THE DOCTOR'S GUIDE TO

SLEEP SOLUTIONS
FOR STRESS & ANXIETY

D1405541

THE DOCTOR'S GUIDE TO

SLEEP SOLUTIONS FOR STRESS & ANXIETY

COMBAT STRESS AND SLEEP EASIER EVERY NIGHT

ROBERT S. ROSENBERG, D.O., F.C.C.P.

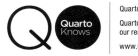

Quarto is the authority on a wide range of topics.

Quarto educates, entertains and enriches the lives of our readers—enthusiasts and lovers of hands-on living.

www.QuartoKnows.com

First published in the United States of America in 2016 by
Fair Winds Press, an imprint of
Quarto Publishing Group USA Inc.
100 Cummings Center
Suite 406-L
Beverly, Massachusetts 01915-6101
Telephone: (978) 282-9590
Fax: (978) 283-2742
QuartoKnows.com
Visit our blogs at QuartoKnows.com

20 19 18 17 16   1 2 3 4 5

ISBN: 978-1-59233-724-8

Digital edition published in 2016
eISBN: 978-1-63159-169-3
Library of Congress Cataloging-in-Publication Data available.

Design, cover image and page layout: Landers Miller Design
Illustrations: Rick Landers except for 101, 124, 125, 127, 128, 132, and 133 by Gayle Isabelle Ford

Printed in China

The information in this book is for educational purposes only. It is not intended to replace the advice of a physician or medical practitioner. Please see your health-care provider before beginning any new health program.

To my four children,
Jason, Rebecca, Benjamin,
and Matthew Rosenberg,
whom my wife Christine
and I love dearly.

CONTENTS

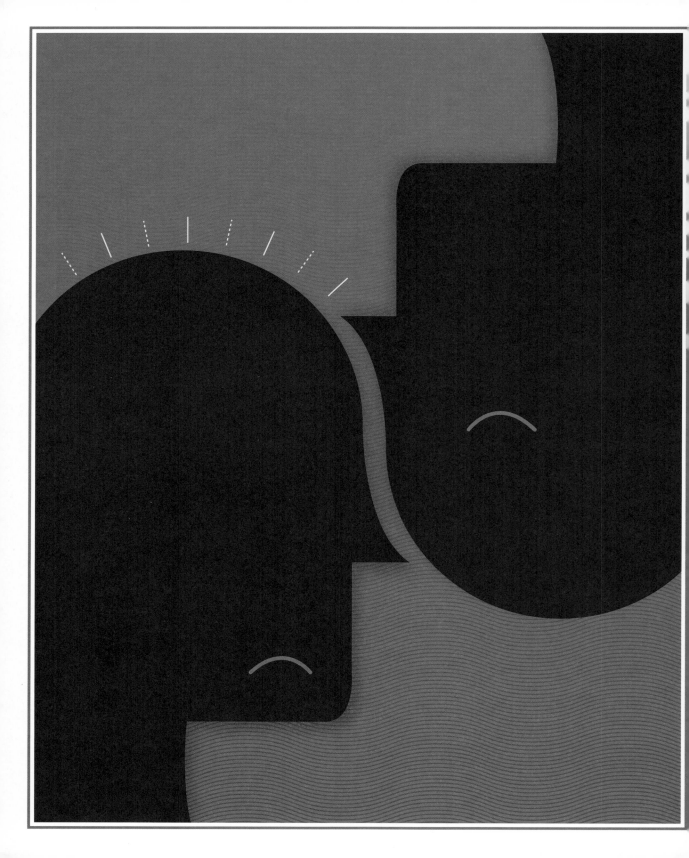

HOW STRESS AND SLEEP ARE LINKED

Tossing and turning at night, especially if something is worrying you, is common. As you watch the hours pass on your bedside clock, your tension increases. You may wake up restless and exhausted, and your energy suffers for the rest of the day.

You are not alone. Insufficient sleep plagues almost half of the global population. You are likely experiencing one of these issues when you try to sleep at night:

- ☽ Too much stress
- ☽ A worried mind
- ☽ A health problem
- ☽ Anxiety
- ☽ Irritation

Think about the stressors in your life right now. Are you dealing with a difficult project at work? Have you been arguing with your spouse? Are you concerned because money is tight? These stressors can prevent you from sleeping and cause you to have fitful nights. Not sleeping also triggers stress hormones and increases your response to minor stressors. You may not notice these ill effects until you eventually become sick, or another health issue crops up.

Disturbed sleep and sleep deprivation worsen stress patterns. They can lead to the common sleep disorder of insomnia, characterized by the inability to fall asleep or stay asleep. People who experience insomnia are rarely able to nap during the day because they are in a state of hyperarousal. In this state, the brain and body do not turn off the fight-or-flight response and they are on constant alert for danger and scanning for threats. Their main symptom is fatigue. Insomnia could come on suddenly and last briefly, or it can become a serious disorder, affecting your ability to think and function well. If not addressed, this persistent sleep disorder negatively affects your mood, mental function, and overall health.

Stress and lack of sleep create a cycle of tension that is hard to break, but there are solutions. This book will explain how stress and anxiety affect your sleeping, eating, emotional health, physical well-being, and mental clarity—and what you can do to overcome them and achieve better sleep. Promise yourself now to choose and apply the best strategies from the book that pertain to you for better sleep and improved health.

How Are Sleep and Stress Linked?

A reciprocal relationship exists between sleep and stress. Someone who is stressed or anxious often has trouble sleeping. However, it works both ways. Those who are sleep deprived will often have problems dealing with minor stressors. In one study, the subjects, when sleep deprived, perceived and reacted to minor stressors the same way they responded to major stressors. At the same time, a control group, which had slept eight hours, did not react appreciably to the minor stressors used in the study.

What we learn from the study is that sleep deprivation lowers our psychological threshold for how we perceive and react to stress. In brain studies that use functional MRIs, we see increased brain activity based on the blood flow to a particular brain region. When conducted after a night of fewer than six hours of sleep, we see hyperactivity in the emotional brain center called the amygdala. (See how the amygdala influences your emotions on page 54.) At the same time, there is decreased blood flow to the higher cortical brain centers responsible for executive thinking skills and control of our emotions. The amygdala's normal inhibition that exists after a good night's sleep is absent. Thus, we overreact psychologically in the form of fear and anxiety. We overreact physically as well with symptoms like rapid heartbeat, shortness of breath, or excessive sweating to stimuli that normally would not elicit much of a reaction at all.

The connections between stressors and sleep are in your biochemistry. Lack of sleep triggers a stress response, which has three phases, and these can be caused by lack of sleep but also by other stressors.

① The first phase is the initial activation of the sympathetic nervous system that increases your heart rate, blood pressure, and breathing. Adrenaline production increases to give you an energy edge to escape danger.

② Once the activation settles a bit, the second phase refers to how you adapt. That is, how are you emotionally after stress activation? How soon can you get back to normal? In short, are you a resilient person?

③ The third phase is fatigue and overtiredness. You become exhausted, and this is when the stress turns chronic. The good news is that you can get control before excess stress makes you feel out of control.

Stress is a common experience for people, but most people don't know how stress affects them and how to get help. Most people can't see clearly how the lack of sleep and stress overload are connected. Together, the patterns can destabilize energy, focus, and mood. One patient of mine, Karen, explained her sleep issue to me after her husband urged her to consult with a sleep professional. Karen described the scene clearly:

I am awake early, like 3:30 or 4 a.m., and just being in bed wanting to sleep is really irritating, so I get up. I know I am not going back to bed, so I use the treadmill, feed the cats, and start cooking for the day. An aroma of onions and garlic fills the house, and my husband George comes into the kitchen.

"Honey," he says, "Are you okay?"

I turn on him with a vengeance. "You know I can't sleep. Damn it! No, I am not okay. I'm exhausted. Every time I get up early, you ask me that stupid question."

"Geez. I'm sorry, and I'm going back to bed."

"No you're not," I commanded him like an infantry sergeant. "You are going to walk that poor dog that never gets outside anymore. Why don't you get some exercise?"

Karen's husband asked her to consult with me after this incident. My diagnosis for Karen was insomnia, and she was committed to having better sleep habits and gaining control of her angry outbursts. I saw Karen again about six months later, and her story had a very different tone.

"You know, Dr. Rosenberg, I had no idea how horrible I was acting toward my husband, and even toward my oldest son. When I was angry all the time, I knew that I was acting out, but I was also in a fog. I couldn't control the

CHECK-IN:
HOW IS YOUR STRESS LEVEL?

Why not check in with yourself now? Add a checkmark beside any of the following events you have experienced consistently over the past two weeks:

○ You don't seem able to relax.

○ You have been overwhelmed with responsibilities.

○ You have had difficulty getting to sleep.

○ You have had trouble staying asleep.

○ You can't stop worrying about responsibilities.

You are experiencing stress if you checked three or more items. The more items you checked, the more difficult your stress could be. See page 77 to learn more about stress resolutions.

○ You have felt irritated, short-tempered, or crabby.

○ You have lost your motivation to finish tasks or projects.

○ You have been sick or had problems getting over an illness.

○ You use a substance (alcohol or others) to relax so you can sleep.

outbursts and I didn't care about whom my action affected.

"Now that my sleeping has improved so well, I get up in the morning, and I am happy. I don't get mad at the dog. Instead, I take her for a walk. I make breakfast, and George and I have some time to share conversation before he heads out the door. Even my son noted how I was smiling for a change. It is nice to be me again."

Karen's story portrayed the difference in her personality when she went from poor sleep to

sleeping six or more hours a night. However, I think her hard-learned lesson was taking back control of her stress reactions and moodiness that pushed the people she loved away from her.

Good stress (called eustress) is a positive motivator and helps you move forward. In this case, you are most likely sleeping deeply and at least seven to nine hours. Your brain and body are repairing and balancing all systems while you sleep.

The more positive forms of stress are associated with getting your first car, graduating from college, having wonderful relationships, having a child, or moving into a new home. The not-so-positive forms of stress, such as those that nibbled away at Karen's resilience, include job demands and financial problems. The next section explains how stress overload eroded Karen's resilience, causing her to worry at night and lose sleep until she was in distress and felt out of control.

When Karen was able to retrain her sleep habits, she took back control of the runaway stress reactions. She regained a sense of self-esteem, as sleep healed Karen's stress response process. This book will help you get your stress and anxiety under control, as Karen has, and finally sleep better.

How Stress Affects Sleep

Stress is a primary contributor to sleep disorders such as insomnia. And vice versa—sleep disorders can cause and exacerbate stress, anxiety, and other mental health issues. How you react to stress psychologically and physically affects how you

TERM REVIEW

Sleep professionals define insomnia as difficulty falling asleep (sleep onset), trouble staying asleep (sleep maintenance), or waking earlier than your normal waking schedule. These three types of insomnia are characterized by the duration of the symptoms.

Transient insomnia has a brief duration up to several days because a life circumstance may cause stress and then the circumstance is over.

Chronic insomnia is defined as occurring at least three nights a week and endures for one month or longer.

Cognitive intrusions are repetitive images, thoughts, or impulses that interrupt your sleep or another activity. They are difficult to control or "turn off" when trying to fall asleep.

Good stress (called eustress) is a positive motivator and helps you move forward.

sleep. A sudden event, such as the loss of a loved one or an auto accident, or longer-term stressors, such as financial pressures or chronic illness, can lead to transient or chronic insomnia.

People with chronic insomnia are ill prepared to deal with stress. They are more prone to ruminating and suffer frequent cognitive intrusions, especially around bedtime. They have difficulty falling asleep and staying asleep. When they see a sleep professional, their classic complaints are that they cannot shut their mind down, thoughts keep turning in their heads, and they cannot stop worrying.

Why is this? Insomnia causes elevated cortisol and adrenaline production. Elevated cortisol depresses deep slow-wave sleep and also causes fatigue and loss of concentration, inhibits memory consolidation, and depresses immunity. People experience an overproduction of stress hormones such as cortisol and adrenaline that predisposes them to stress-induced insomnia. Their symptoms typically include an overactive sympathetic (fight-or-flight) nervous system as well as: a hyperactive HPA (hypothalamic-pituitary-adrenal) axis, resulting in the overproduction of stress hormones; and severely impaired and disrupted sleep. More important, increasing cortisol can negatively affect receptors in the brain for the neurotransmitters serotonin, dopamine, and norepinephrine, all of which play a prominent role in regulating sleep as well as our emotional reactions.

The results are poor sleep and poor sleep behaviors. People with insomnia often relapse when they stop taking sleeping pills. They are still unequipped to deal with the underlying problem of stress. Given solid nights of sleep, the brain and body heal and restore physiological systems.

How Interrupted Sleep Affects Mood

Pay attention to your moods. Do your moods stay even throughout the day, or do they fluctuate? The amount of your uninterrupted sleep has an effect on your moods.

Take Elena, an attorney for a large corporation, for example. At the end of her workday, she arrived home to her five-month-old son, his nanny, and Joe, her husband. Joe is also a lawyer and worked part time for a non-profit organization. She tended to her son during the night if he cried out, and this interrupted her sleep. Elena wasn't sleeping well and experienced up-and-down mood cycles throughout the day. Her physician referred her to my sleep clinic.

New parents typically find their sleep disrupted for five or ten minutes several times during the night. In a recent survey, 20 percent of parents of newborn to three-year-olds reported waking up three or more times per night on average. This type of interrupted sleep can be difficult to change, so it's important to understand the effects.

Researchers set out to find the consequences of such sleep disruptions and how they affect

DEBUNKING THE "CATCHING UP ON SLEEP" MYTH

Usually, how many hours of sleep do you get at night?

1942	1942	1990	2001	2004	2013
	%	%	%	%	%
Five or fewer hours	3	14	16	14	14
Six hours	8	28	27	26	26
Seven hours	25	30	28	28	25
Eight hours	45	22	24	25	29
Nine or more hours	14	5	4	6	5
NET: Six or fewer hours	11	42	43	40	40
NET: Seven or more hours	84	57	56	59	59
Average hours per night	7.9	6.7	6.7	6.8	6.8

The Gallup Poll shows that 40 percent of Americans are sleeping six hours or less at night. Although 59 percent of Americans are sleeping seven hours or more according to this poll, the average night's sleep is still almost an hour less than that of the people surveyed in 1942.

The relationship between sleep and brain function is simple. For the brain to function, you need good-quality sleep. Studies show that poor-quality sleep can damage or destroy brain cells. In one study, prolonged wakefulness in mice is linked to loss of neurons in a critical area of the brain called the locus coeruleus (LC). The LC is vital for alertness and cognition. Researchers then observed mice after periods of normal sleep, short wakefulness, or extended wakefulness. After several days of extended wakefulness, the mice exhibited a 25 percent loss of neurons in the LC. A protein called SIRT3, which protects brain cells from oxidative stress and death, was depleted. However, after short periods of sleep loss with normal amounts of sleep, the levels of SIRT3 increased and were protective.

For years, we assumed that cognitive abilities recover after short- and long-term sleep loss. However, this study demonstrates that brain cells can be damaged or can die from prolonged periods of insufficient sleep, leading to permanent cognitive dysfunction. These findings also debunk the myth that you can catch up on your sleep on your days off or on the weekend, because brain cell damage may have already occurred and is not so easily reversed.

As of now, more than 33 percent of the population admits to sleeping less than seven hours per night; many of them sleep less than five. Moreover, the percentage of the population getting adequate sleep has decreased over time, as shown in the chart above. The mice study shows what a high price these people pay for not getting seven to nine hours of quality sleep each night, and there is no "catching up."

Jones, Jeffrey M. "In the U.S., 40% Get Less Than Recommended Amount of Sleep." www.gallup.com/poll/166553/less-recommended-amount-sleep.aspx.

mood or the ability to maintain attention and alertness over prolonged periods. Students with no prior sleep problems took tests to gauge moods and maintain focus one hour after waking. They performed under three different conditions.

They were tested first after eight hours of uninterrupted sleep. The next set of tests was after sleep was restricted to four hours. The last test occurred after a night in which they were awakened for ten minutes after every ninety minutes of sleep.

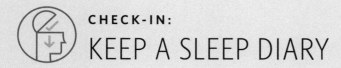

KEEP A SLEEP DIARY

Keeping a sleep diary can help determine the reasons you have problems sleeping. A sleep diary helps you keep track of behaviors and habits that interfere with sleep, and it will help you identify any problems. Take five to ten minutes a day to fill in your patterns, and a sleep diary will help you and your doctor reach a diagnosis and solutions faster.

7 p.m.	I played with my son, gave him a bath, and put him down to sleep.
7:45 to 9 p.m.	I worked on my legal cases.
9 p.m.	Joe and I relaxed with a glass or two of wine and retired to our bedroom. We read or talked and turned out the light. Then I became irritated because I knew the baby would wake me eventually and I would have trouble getting to sleep again.
10 p.m.	I was still awake.
10:35 p.m.	I attended to my son and returned to sleep.
12 a.m.	I went to the bathroom. I checked on my son, who was asleep.
1 a.m.	I returned to sleep.
3:15 a.m.	I attended to my son and returned to sleep.
4:30 a.m.	I was awake again and irritated.
5:30 a.m.	I never returned to sleep. I tryed to stay in bed until 6 or 6:30 a.m., and was not successful. I got out of bed. I was out the door and on my way to work at 7:30 a.m.

MEASURE MOODS AND SLEEP

Keeping track of both sleep and moodiness are barometers for your well-being. If you want to monitor your sleep patterns and compare those to your moods during the day, start by recording your patterns on the two charts that follow. Be proactive and commit to intentionally designing your sleep and health habits for optimal living.

Mood Diary

Instructions: For each day, circle one number that represents your mood for that day.

Day	Mood	Notes	Overall
		Any events, people, or influences that affected your mood	At the end of the day, which one word describes your mood?
Sunday	① ② ③ ④ ⑤		
Monday	① ② ③ ④ ⑤		
Tuesday	① ② ③ ④ ⑤		
Wednesday	① ② ③ ④ ⑤		
Thursday	① ② ③ ④ ⑤		
Friday	① ② ③ ④ ⑤		
Saturday	① ② ③ ④ ⑤		

Sleep Diary

	Sunday	Monday	Tuesday	Wednesday	Thursday	Friday	Saturday
Time I went to bed							
Time I got up in the morning							
I woke up X times at night							
Number of hours I slept							

During this ten-minute period, students completed tasks on a computer and returned to sleep.

The results showed that those with interrupted sleep were no better at sustaining attention than those with four hours of sleep. Moodiness, as indicated by depression, fatigue, and reduced energy, increased significantly in those who were restricted to four hours of sleep and those who were awoken for ten minutes every ninety minutes. In summary, brief interruptions of sleep had the same negative impact on mood and consistent attention as a night of severe sleep restriction. In normal sleep patterns, you progress from slow-wave sleep to REM sleep in ninety-minute cycles. If sleep is consistently interrupted, you start again at stage 1 or stage 2, and you may never reach the phase of REM sleep. (See the sleep stages diagram on page 28.)

This study demonstrates the adverse effects of just one night. Imagine the effects of cumulative loss of sleep for shift workers or new parents such as Elena. Sleep disruptions negatively affect their ability to function at the highest level.

I explained to Elena that feeling sleepy during the day, not getting to sleep at night, and waking up feeling exhausted are not typical for the average adult. She thought this was normal for her situation, and she expected to feel tired. She did not expect to be irritable, snappy, teary, and moody, however.

When her doctor referred her to the sleep clinic, Elena thought I would prescribe a medication. She believed she would go home, sleep better, and her moods would change. Her chief complaints were feeling distressed and prone to tears. Most anything irritated her. She seemed tired and always overwrought. She did not know that her prolonged state of hyperarousal drained her energy along with other poor sleep habits.

She filled out several checklists so I could better assess how sleep disturbances influenced moodiness, anxiety, or possible depression (see the Postpartum Depression Checklist on page 147). Elena's score on the General Anxiety Disorder Seven-Item Scale (page 148) indicated that general anxiety was more pronounced than depressive symptoms. I instructed Elena in a plan that included changing her sleep routines for one month. She would keep a sleep diary as well as a moodiness checklist in week four. We could gauge her improvement by less irritability, less moodiness, and better well-being.

She and her husband switched their nightly intake of wine to drinking a choice of sleep-inducing teas. Elena established a calming presleep routine for herself. She kept a regular sleep-wake schedule as best she could, while continuing her sleep diary for the next month. She went to bed when she was truly tired and placed the small alarm clock in the drawer of the nightstand next to the bed. That way she would not be watching the clock but could hear the alarm. Elena began a moderate exercise program on her at-home treadmill. After one month, Elena reported that she felt more energized. She was sleeping better each night and did not feel forgetful each day. Part of the solution involved her husband's involvement in co-parenting and assisting with their son when he was awake at intervals through the night.

Elena's story demonstrates how sleep entwines with moods. Inadequate sleep contributes to negative moods such as feeling cranky, annoyed, grumpy, nervous, tense, or worried. Likewise, quality sleep promotes better moods such as feeling happy, energetic, calm, refreshed, or playful.

Average Sleep Time versus Ideal Sleep Time by Country

Stress, everyday schedules and routines, and work affect sleep time. These variables differ across different countries and cultures. A 2013 National Sleep Foundation study found that significant differences in sleep behavior exist among participants in the six countries studied. Some additional noteworthy findings from this study include the following:

》 Americans and Japanese report significantly less sleep on workdays than do other countries.

》 Mexican participants reported requiring the most sleep (8 hours, 15 minutes).

》 Roughly one-half of respondents from the United States and Japan had taken naps in the past two weeks.

》 About 9 in 10 Mexicans reported they slept through the night at least a few nights a week. One-third or more of participants in the United States, United Kingdom, and Germany said they rarely or never slept through the night in the past two weeks.

》 Respondents from Japan are more likely to sleep alone. Those from the United States are more likely to sleep with pets.

》 Thirty percent of respondents in the United Kingdom sleep wearing nothing most nights (compared to 0 to 14 percent in other countries).

Average Sleep Time versus Ideal Sleep Time by Country

Country	Average time slept work nights	Average sleep needed to function best	Participants who got a good night's sleep most nights	Participants whose schedule allows adequate sleep
United States	6 hours, 31 minutes	7 hours, 13 minutes	44 percent	72 percent
Canada	7 hours, 3 minutes	7 hours, 22 minutes	43 percent	70 percent
Mexico	7 hours, 6 minutes	8 hours, 15 minutes	48 percent	66 percent
United Kingdom	6 hours, 49 minutes	7 hours, 20 minutes	42 percent	82 percent
Germany	7 hours, 1 minute	7 hours, 31 minutes	40 percent	72 percent
Japan	6 hours, 22 minutes	6 hours, 58 minutes	54 percent	66 percent

» All (100 percent) of the German respondents air out their bedroom once per week. Fresh air was very important to German respondents as compared to participants in other countries.

» Having a pleasant scent in the bedroom was very important to Mexican respondents as compared to participants in other countries.

Stress Less, Sleep Better

The information in this section can be alarming, especially if you have suffered from insomnia for a while. There is good news, however. Given solid nights of sleep, the brain and body can heal and restore these imbalanced physiological processes.

But strong coping skills are crucial. You can foster better coping skills right away by getting regular daily exercise; incorporating more nutritional foods into your diet; and eliminating nicotine, caffeine, and other stimulants. The most important coping skill you need to master, though, is how you deal with stress. Learn to manage your stress before it turns into excessive worry, anxiety, or panic. In the chapters that follow, you'll read about many strategies that help reduce anxiety levels and intrusive thoughts, including cognitive behavioral therapy for insomnia, meditation, and hypnosis.

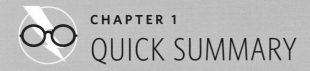

CHAPTER 1

QUICK SUMMARY

» Stress and sleep are closely linked. Stress overload is debilitating and can disrupt sleep. Likewise, lack of sleep inhibits your neurobiology to repair any damage or consolidate learning and memory. This mix can lead to insomnia—your inability to get to sleep, stay asleep, or wake up refreshed because you are in a state of hyperarousal.

» The three levels of stress responses feed off of each other. Most people are not aware that stress, when not accounted for or managed, can escalate to distress.

» Without healthy sleep, the hyperarousal state becomes your new normal. Poor sleep and stress need prompt attention.

CHAPTER 2

THE BENEFITS OF SLEEP AND THE DANGERS OF INSUFFICIENT SLEEP

Good-quality sleep that lasts seven to nine hours has unparalleled benefits for physical health: It supports a strong immune system, good memory, and better focus. Your emotions are better balanced. Healthy sleep regulates your appetite efficiently. High-quality sleep is also key in treating stress and anxiety. Although you may not be aware, lack of sleep can cause negative and stressful responses to completely neutral stimuli, such as a facial expression or even a kind word. Let's look at the benefits of high-quality sleep first.

Benefits of Sleep

You know you feel better after a good night's sleep, but there are more benefits than you may realize.

Strong Immune System

We know that sleep is necessary for your immune system to function normally, and research supports that our immune system works best when we get adequate sleep. People who are sleep deprived demonstrate poor responses (lower antibody response) to vaccines for influenza and hepatitis, studies show. They mount a delayed and lowered antibody response to a vaccine that produces antibodies that attack the virus or bacteria. This response can be insufficient when a person is sleep deprived. When you are sick or have an infection, the need to sleep and get well is also the body's natural intuition. Sleeping during and even after infections promotes healing and strength rebuilding.

Emotional Well-Being

Chronically sleep-deprived individuals have a higher incidence of anxiety disorders and depression. Sleep plays a critical role in emotional processing, which takes place in great part during the REM sleep stage, but is not confined to this stage of sleep.

There is a clear relationship between insomnia and depression, as indicated by the 90 percent of patients diagnosed with major depression who also report sleep disturbances. Chronic insomnia often predates depression by years.

It is important to know that if one suffers from depression and the insomnia is not treated, it tends to persist. As a result, the rate of relapse of depression is high.

There are several ways to address insomnia and depression. Cognitive behavioral therapy for insomnia (CBTI) techniques combine behavioral modifications with strategies to eliminate dysfunctional beliefs about sleep. If you use medications, some sedating antidepressant medications can treat the depression and insomnia at the same time. Sleep medications such as zolpidem and eszopiclone have been found effective in some studies when given in concert with standard antidepressants for a short period of time. The results are even better in conjunction with sleep hygiene and cognitive behavioral therapies.

Brain Health

Our brains perform several regenerative processes at night while we sleep. The process, referred to as neuroplasticity, occurs when the brain forms new neural pathways and connections, and this happens predominantly during sleep. Moreover, neurobiological cleaning chores, such as clearing out various neurotoxins that build up during the day, happen ten times faster during sleep. The brain also replenishes its energy sources in the form of the molecule adenosine triphosphate (ATP) while we sleep.

Tissue Repair and Growth

Most of our growth hormone production occurs during sleep, is closely linked to deep or slow-wave sleep, and is especially important during children's growth years. In adults, this process repairs tissue, muscle, and bone and is critical for new cell formation. Enough sleep is essential in helping your musculoskeletal system restore itself, especially for bodybuilders and athletes. If you are a postmenopausal woman, insufficient sleep can predispose you to osteoporosis.

Healthy Weight Maintenance

If you want to lose weight and reduce your waistline, then you have to get seven to nine hours of sleep each night and burn calories with exercise. Insufficient sleep leads to excessive production of a hormone called ghrelin, which promotes appetite. Have you observed that if you don't sleep well one night, you seem overly hungry the next day? Insufficient sleep also impedes production of the appetite-suppressing hormone leptin. Think of the implications for college students and young adults who spend long night hours studying, partying, or working. This is also why we see a much higher

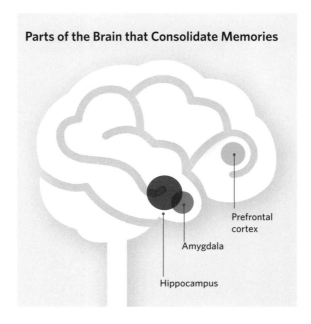

Parts of the Brain that Consolidate Memories

Prefrontal cortex

Amygdala

Hippocampus

> Sleep-deprived individuals remember predominantly negative and anxiety-provoking images the following day to the exclusion of positive memories.

incidence of obesity in shift workers who commonly get no more than six hours of sleep a night.

Longer Life Span

If you chronically sleep fewer than seven hours, you are more likely to develop hypertension, stroke, or heart attack. As a result, you have a shorter life span.

Memory Consolidation

Sleep is necessary for memory consolidation. There are two broad types of memories. Declarative memory is expressed verbally and involves the learning of factual material and remembering the order of episodes in our lives. Procedural memory refers to recalling how to ride a bike, drive a car, or play an instrument. When people get a good night's sleep after learning new information, they perform better on testing than those who do not sleep well.

Sleep more efficiently consolidates our emotional, impactful events rather than neutral events. Whether those memories are negative or positive doesn't matter. When sleep deprived, we tend to consolidate more negative memories of the day. In studies, sleep-deprived individuals remembered predominantly negative and anxiety-provoking images the following day to the exclusion of positive memories.

Memory consolidation works like this: First, your brain's hippocampus uploads short-term, unstable information packets plus experiences. Then the brain sends them to the prefrontal cortex, which processes and consolidates the information into more stable and longer lasting memories. This process also involves the amygdala, which stores emotional memories. It is interesting that we tend to preferentially consolidate and remember memories attached to strong emotions.

The prefrontal cortex is also instrumental in a process called fear extinction memory, where very negative conditioned memories in the amygdala are replaced by more positive ones. If you are sleep deprived, this is unlikely to occur, and so your negative memories remain stronger.

The Dangers of Insufficient Sleep

Remember these two significant results each time you make a decision to skip sleep, stay up later, or complain about how you feel during the day. First, disrupted sleep can result in damage to your genes, which explains how people develop infections and disease through an impaired immune function. This happens because lack of sleep causes the release of inflammatory mediators, and, at the same time, sets off a process called oxidative stress, which can be highly damaging to our DNA. Second, lack of healthy sleep affects the brain and changes how you function during the day. You might make poor decisions while sleep deprived. You might feel fatigued and overreact emotionally. When this happens, you have to ask yourself whether lack of sleep and the results are worth such risks. Let's look at each of these processes.

Poor Immune System Function

The adage "Early to bed, early to rise makes a man healthy, wealthy, and wise" has some truth to it. We recognize now how insufficient sleep affects our immune system. Studies over the past twenty years clearly demonstrate this relationship. A report titled *Prospective Study of Sleep Duration and Pneumonia Risk in Women* showed how inadequate sleep increased the risk of pneumonia by 40 percent. Sleep directly affects your ability to cope with and prevent infection. Sleep is as important to your health and well-being as food, fresh air, and water.

We produce peripheral blood mononuclear cells (PBMC), which are essential for the production of infection-fighting antibodies, during sleep. Also during sleep, your body produces proteins called cytokines that not only fight infection but also help regulate sleep. There are many types of cytokines, some inflammatory and some anti-inflammatory. With insufficient sleep, we increase the production of the cytokines that promote inflammation. The cytokines called interleukin-6 (IL-6) can cross the blood–brain barrier and increase the release of stress hormones, which negatively affect sleep and hinder your immune system.

Risk of Diabetes

There is a clear relationship between insufficient sleep and the incidence of diabetes. Sleeping six hours or less each night can cause a craving for high-calorie carbohydrates. These cravings, combined with a slower metabolism and elevated cortisol levels resulting from sleep deprivation, cause you to gain weight. Weight gain leads your body to develop resistance to insulin, which leads to diabetes.

Living with diabetes creates additional health problems, including poor sleep, especially if you don't manage your condition properly. Diabetes can contribute to and possibly cause sleep apnea, a condition in which you experience pauses in air intake or shallow breathing during sleep, causing you to wake frequently. This may be due to nerve damage from chronically elevated blood sugar. It is speculated that this may be the basis of the inordinately high incidence of sleep apnea in diabetics. However, the reverse is also true: Sleep apnea can lead to diabetes by causing insulin resistance and depressing insulin production by the pancreas.

Insufficient sleep or a circadian disorder called shift workers' disorder can predispose you to diabetes. The body's internal clock is closely tied to bodily functions such as glucose metabolism. One study shows that the pancreas contains receptors for melatonin, a sleep-regulating hormone that is also necessary for normal insulin production.

If you live with diabetes or have a higher risk because of poor sleep, you can improve your health with natural solutions that allow you to rest easier. Focus on eating a balanced, nutritious diet low in processed foods to give your body a metabolism boost and the energy it needs during the day. (For nutrition suggestions, see page 91.) To help your internal clock recognize when it is time to sleep, begin a daily exercise routine so that you are able to get more fulfilling rest later on. (See chapter 13 for exercise and movement suggestions.)

Sleep Debt and Anxiety

Not sleeping enough for multiple days in a row is known as sleep debt. It can cause anxiety or make your current anxiety symptoms worse.

Two weeks of less than six hours of sleep at night decreases alertness and performance equivalent to a complete twenty-four hours of sleep deprivation. One week of just four hours of sleep at night amounts two to three days with no sleep. Lack of focus and efficiency during the day continues and strengthens as sleep debt develops. Sleep debt can increase body stress to a point of dysfunction because the lack of sleep disrupts neurons from their usual repair functions. For example, the temporal lobe, which handles auditory functions and language, becomes limited due to neuronal damage when the brain doesn't get enough sleep. Likewise, a lack of sleep elevates levels of cortisol and adrenaline, leading to hyperarousal.

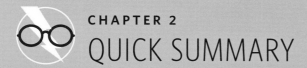

CHAPTER 2

QUICK SUMMARY

» Healthy sleep supports a strong immune system and allows the time and space for your brain and body to make necessary repairs.

» Sleep also plays a critical role in processing emotions. If you aren't sleeping, you may experience your emotional reactions as more dramatic or overt. Your thinking may become more negative. Chronic insomnia usually predates developing depression. Both persist if not treated. Treat poor sleep promptly.

» Irritability, moodiness, fatigue, fuzzy thinking, and headaches also result from lost sleep.

CHAPTER 3

A HEALTHY SLEEP CYCLE

You need to make sleep a priority, as there is no true substitute for the health benefits and prevention of further health problems. Sleep is one of your best tools for healthy living and is necessary for your emotional and physical well-being. If you also have trouble seeing the bigger picture of how stress affects your sleep and health, then a portrait of healthy sleep is where to start.

Sleep is the foundation of your health, and you need seven to nine hours of sleep each night to repair stressed systems. You wake up from this type of sleep feeling revitalized. How long you sleep is important because sleep cycles through four stages. Each stage is deeper than the first because certain maintenance activities happen within each stage.

The ability to reach and sustain uninterrupted REM sleep and deep sleep is necessary for dreaming and for the brain to consolidate what you learned into memory and process emotions. If you wake up before entering the deeper stages of sleep, your body starts over again at either stage 1 or 2, which are the lighter and less restorative stages of sleep.

Sleep Architecture

The word *architecture* refers to the process and the product of a design. Sleep architecture describes the process of sleep as well as the end results. The process of sleep architecture is a ninety-minute repeating cycle through the two main types of sleep, non-rapid eye movement (NREM) and rapid eye movement (REM). The product of sleep architecture is seven to nine hours of sleep, which promotes full restoration and good health.

You need to sleep long enough (sleep duration) and deeply enough (sleep depth) to allow for the body's normal repair functions. These functions are a vital part of the sleep stages, as each stage fulfills its role in preparing you for the next day.

"Arousals" refer to when you wake up in the middle of the night, or you are aware of changing positions and then go back to sleep. You experience partial arousals if you are not very awake and have no recollection of them in the morning. On the other hand, you may not wake up at all during these subcortical arousals that manifest as spikes in blood pressure and heart rate, but are not discernable even on a simultaneously recorded EEG. You will realize the importance of arousals in further discussions of how sleep is disrupted and how stress results.

In normal sleep, you go to bed and move through sleep stages from wakefulness to lighter sleep, to deeper sleep (slow-wave sleep), to REM sleep. This cycle repeats throughout the night with REM predominating in the second half of the night. This baseline is a useful way to gauge how you sleep.

NREM sleep includes three stages of sleep, or 75 percent of the night. Each stage of NREM sleep is deeper than the previous one.

The Four Stages of Sleep

The four stages of sleep, a repeating ninety-minute cycle, promote restoration and both mental and physical repair.

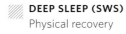

DEEP SLEEP (SWS)
Physical recovery

DREAMING (REM)
Mental recovery

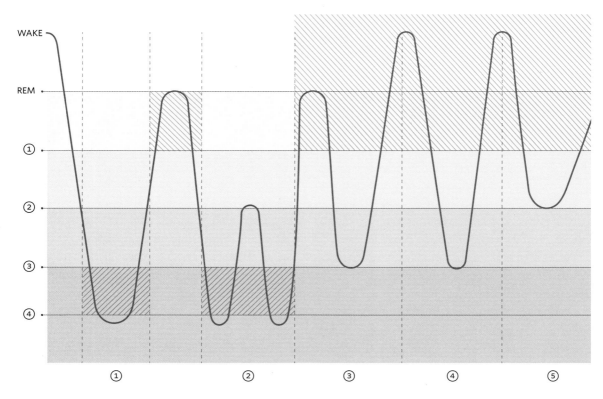

Source: Adapted from the National Institutes of Health.

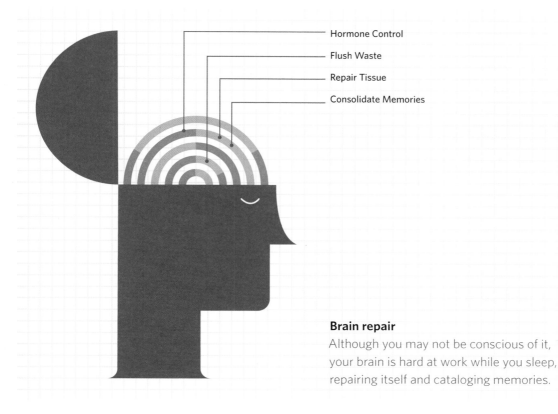

Hormone Control

Flush Waste

Repair Tissue

Consolidate Memories

Brain repair
Although you may not be conscious of it, your brain is hard at work while you sleep, repairing itself and cataloging memories.

Stage 1 is shallow sleep or light sleep and occurs from 2 to 5 percent of nightly sleep. If you have trouble going to sleep and spend more time in stage 1, you have disturbed sleep, not restful sleep. When you are not falling asleep, most likely you are worried, restless, or ruminating.

Stage 2 is when you sleep. Body temperature drops and breathing is regular and decreased.

Stage 3 is deeper sleep, which activates restoration of muscles, tissue repair, circulation, and energy.

REM sleep refers to rapid eye movement sleep, the last stage in which most but not all dreaming takes place. REM cycling begins about ninety minutes into sleep. As it recurs throughout the night, each cycle becomes progressively longer. The limbs become still like a kind of paralysis.

Almost all muscles, except the diaphragm and eye muscles, become much weaker. The brain is active in dreaming and learning consolidation, especially emotionally laden memories. The body gains energy to support you through the day.

I cannot emphasize enough how uninterrupted sleep of a seven to nine hours maintains good health and improves emotional stability and mental functions. Throughout the sleep stages, the brain and body make repairs such as controlling appetite hormones, flushing waste matter from the brain, repairing tissue, and consolidating memories of what you learned that day.

Circadian Rhythms

Like all creatures on planet Earth, humans evolved within a cycle of light and dark, day and

Circadian Rythems

Your body prepares for sleep even while you are awake or while addressing your other physical and mental needs.

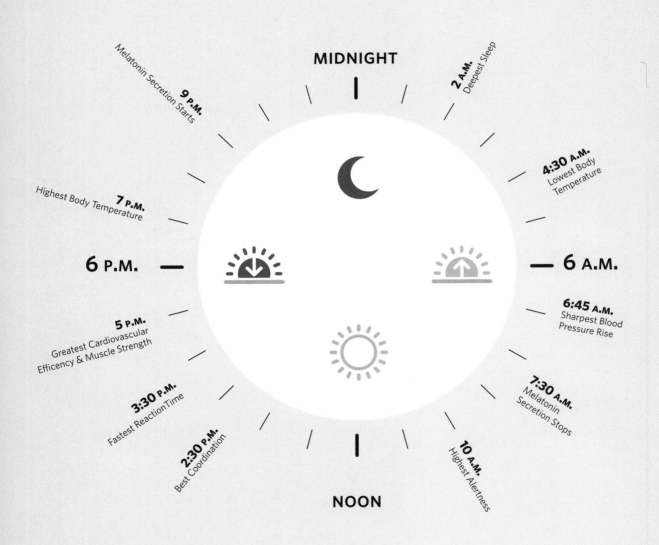

MIDNIGHT

9 P.M. Melatonin Secretion Starts

2 A.M. Deepest Sleep

4:30 A.M. Lowest Body Temperature

7 P.M. Highest Body Temperature

6 P.M.

6 A.M.

6:45 A.M. Sharpest Blood Pressure Rise

5 P.M. Greatest Cardiovascular Efficency & Muscle Strength

7:30 A.M. Melatonin Secretion Stops

3:30 P.M. Fastest Reaction Time

2:30 P.M. Best Coordination

10 A.M. Highest Alertness

NOON

night, as determined by the rising and setting of the sun. Your biology is normally in accord with the natural twenty-four- to twenty-five-hour cycle that regulates eating, sleeping, and other activities. Your biological clock responds to light by waking up and to darkness by going to sleep. However, we often override the decision to sleep. Or other factors such as stress, worry, or anxiety keep us awake, and we miss the benefits of the reparation. If your sleep schedule changes and you wake up during the night, you disrupt your inner clock.

The primary circadian rhythm within the brain modulates body temperature, muscle tone, heart rate, and much of hormonal secretion. When your rhythm is disrupted, you may experience

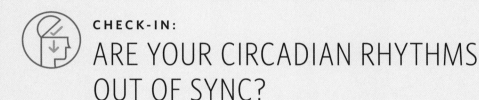

CHECK-IN:

ARE YOUR CIRCADIAN RHYTHMS OUT OF SYNC?

Our master clock runs every cell, hormone, and function of the body. If circadian rhythms are dysregulated, we feel out of control and out of time. How do you function?

The characteristics below (even just one of these symptoms) are indicative that you are out of sync with your internal biorhythms. You are more likely to experience some disorder in eating, feeling, thinking, or sleeping.

① You don't get much sunlight.

② You wake up at night.

③ You have trouble going to sleep.

④ You experience sadness or depression in the winter.

⑤ You are irritable during the day.

⑥ You have mood swings.

⑦ You feel dull and slow.

⑧ You can be oversensitive to environmental stimuli such as loud sounds.

delayed sleep, hormone dysregulation, and changes in body temperature and mood. Not sleeping disrupts the circadian master clock, also called the suprachiasmatic nucleus (SCN), a region of the hypothalamus. This daily cycle controls more than just the sleep-wake cycles. Each organ and body function has its own rhythm and schedule.

Our optimal physical health, emotional balance, and good mood depend on stable circadian rhythms or sleep cycles. You might have experienced disrupted rhythms if you had jet lag or worked a night shift schedule. You disrupt the circadian clocks to your detriment when you deprive yourself of sleep. You need deep, slow-wave, and REM sleep to repair and rebalance the brain and body. In REM sleep, the neurotransmitters serotonin and norepinephrine can turn off and rest. In fact, they are at their lowest levels during REM sleep. Turning off returns sensitivity levels to receptors for norepinephrine and serotonin and allows other neurotransmitters to stay at normal levels. Moods improve and your ability to learn increases. Staying regulated through sleep lets regular healing takes place and enhances your mental and emotional health.

With disrupted circadian rhythms, you may experience certain symptoms. If your body produces melatonin during the day instead of at night, you might feel as Karen did and experience dullness and irritability. You could experience a lapse of good judgment and make more mistakes because you are not alert. Low energy could feel like exhaustion, lethargy, or dullness. Depression can also result.

Mobile Sleep Apps

If you are interested in tracking your sleep with mobile apps, you should be aware of what they can and cannot provide. Sleep apps can give you a reasonable estimation of your time asleep based on readings from an accelerometer. This device reads and interprets movement that indicates you are awake, and lack of movement indicates you are asleep. They tend to overestimate sleep by as much as 30 to 45 minutes, because sometimes we lie still when awake. The apps may pick up movement of a bed partner and interpret it as wakefulness. They are also somewhat dependent on the material of the mattress or pillow to transmit vibrations. Activity and fitness trackers worn on the wrist are likely to offer better readings.

Beware of apps that claim to tell you what stages of sleep you are in during the night or claim to have an alarm that will go off as you transition to light sleep in the morning. When studied in sleep laboratories with simultaneous EEG tracings, they have been found to be off significantly when discerning different stages of sleep.

In my own practice, I have used them with my insomnia patients as a complement to sleep diaries when I am tracking my patient's response to therapy. I use them to give me a general idea of how long it takes the patient to fall asleep and the approximate length of sleep.

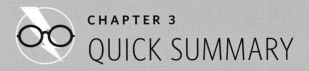

CHAPTER 3
QUICK SUMMARY

» Sleep architecture is the pattern of sleep that alternates between NREM sleep and REM sleep. During deep sleep, repair functions include tissue growth, renewing energy, and release of essential growth hormone.

» Restorative sleep repairs and balances neurobiological rhythms, including healthy immune function, appetite regulation, repair of stressed systems, and memory consolidation.

» Sleep cycles affect the depth of sleep and the duration of sleep. The deepest sleep is slow-wave, which produces twice the restorative effect as lighter stages of sleep do.

» REM sleep is critical in processing emotions and consolidating certain types of memory, and thus is important in dealing with stress.

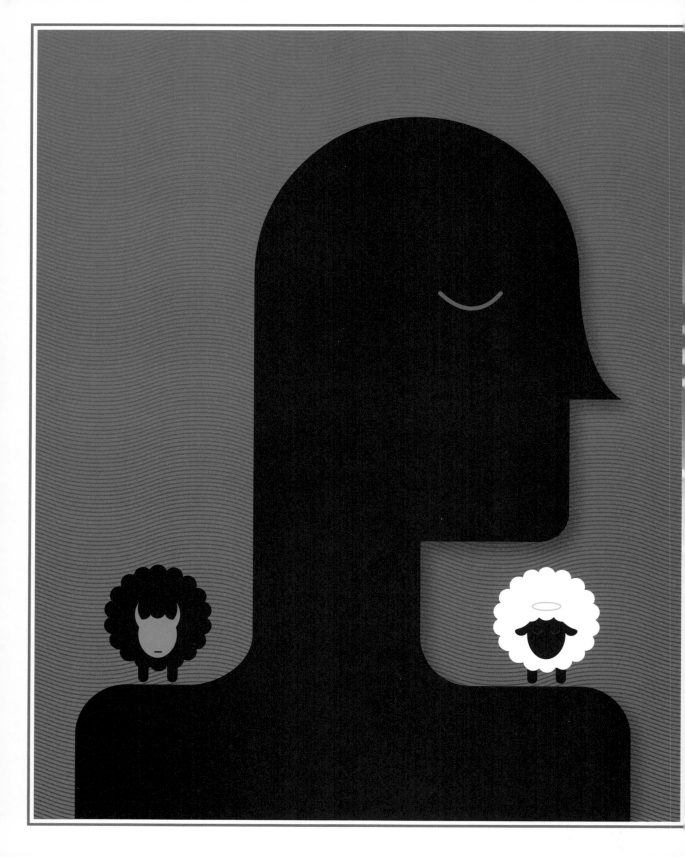

CHAPTER 4

CREATE GOOD HABITS AND AVOID BAD HABITS

Your commitment to sleep means changing your environment and limiting what appears or happens in your bedroom to only that which promotes sleep. Clear any clutter of books, magazines, electronic gadgets, and computers. Move the television out of the bedroom. The purpose here is to train your brain to pick up new habits that support your quality of sleep.

The best way to do this is to eliminate the competition to your sleep. That could be what you ingest or what you read or watch. In addition to the elimination checklists that appear in this chapter, I suggest you not sleep with pets or have them in your bedroom at night.

Sleep Hygiene

Sleep hygiene refers to and includes the habits you create for better sleep. Having good-quality sleep requires changing your bedtime surroundings and behaviors that hinder sleep.

Sleep hygiene may resolve sleep issues or lessen their severity, which is why I recommend it as the first steps for patients to implement. Insomnia occurs because your schedule is interrupted and you can't get to sleep, or you

have difficulty staying asleep. Good sleep hygiene restores the order but requires changing your bedtime surroundings and behaviors that hinder sleep. Seven to nine hours of consolidated sleep is your prized ally, and the following suggestions will help you sleep better. To get the best sleep, you need to create an effective sleep environment tailored to your particular needs.

Prepare for Sleeping and Waking Up

Taking a warm bath before bedtime raises your body temperature. Then, exposure to room air after exiting the bath cools you down. A drop in body temperature is a useful signal to the body to enter sleep. Morning sunlight is the cheapest and most widely available sleep aid. Exposure to sunlight within two hours of waking is a strong signal to your circadian clock. It helps you synchronize with your environment and promotes normal sleep time the following night. Sleeping later in the mornings and exposing yourself to light late in the afternoon can desynchronize your internal clock and lead to problems getting up in the morning.

Remember this: Rise at a regular time every day, regardless of the amount of sleep the night before. If you had a bad night and didn't get much sleep, the pressure to sleep the following night will be even greater if you stick to a set wake-up time.

Lighting

Cover windows with dark curtains, shutters, or fabric so that no light shines through and disrupts your sleep. Bright light wakes you up! Red light is the least disturbing to moods and sleep, so if you need a night-light, find one with red bulbs.

Specific cells in the eyes that are susceptible to blue light also regulate your sense of day and night and the seasons. The eyes detect and associate blue light with daylight. Blue light travels via the retinol ganglionic neurons to the hypothalamus, which shuts down the production of melatonin, a sleep-promoting hormone. If your body does not produce melatonin for sleep, and the blue light stimulates you, you are in for a very long night. As for lighting, white low-energy fluorescent and LED bulbs typically produce much more blue light than conventional white incandescent bulbs.

If your livelihood depends on being on computers close to bedtime, look into the software called F.lux. The software turns the color of your electronic device's display to the color of the time of day or evening. An even better option is blue blocker glasses. Although F.lux is great for the background lighting on electronic devices, blue blockers eliminate all sources of blue light at night. They are readily available online.

However, your best bet for limiting blue light is to avoid using electronic devices before bed and while in bed. You can improve your sleep habits simply by turning off computers and smartphones at least one hour before going to bed.

Room Temperature

You'll sleep better in a cooler room than in a warm room because your core body temperature drops at sleep's onset. A room that is too warm inhibits the body's temperature drop, and you'll have a harder time going to sleep. I suggest a room temperature of around 68°F (20°C) because this harmonizes with the drop in body temperature about four to five hours into sleep. The Sleep Foundation discourages temperatures above 75°F (24°C) and below 54°F (12°C), as they will disrupt sleep. If you have a hard time falling asleep, try regulating the room temperature.

Sound

You need a cool, dark, and quiet bedroom for sleeping. If you experience sounds that interfere with sleep, try earplugs or earphones, or use a device that generates white noise or pink noise to even the sound field. If all else fails, the sound of a fan will do the trick.

If your partner's snoring is keeping you awake, you should encourage him or her to be checked by a doctor for sleep apnea. Treatment can improve your health and sleep as well as your partner's sleep.

Alarm Clock

Are you a clock-watcher when you cannot fall or remain asleep? Watching the clock causes two sleep-opposing reactions. The first reaction is calculating time, which results in speeding up your brain waves and making a return to sleep very difficult. The second reaction is provoked anxiety due to mental rumination about how much sleep you will get or how you will function tomorrow. Anxiety and rumination cause the release of stress hormones such as cortisol and adrenaline, which normally are at their lowest levels during sleep. Rumination then makes it difficult to return to sleep and impossible for the body to reduce stress hormones and restore balance. Place your alarm clock somewhere you cannot see it, such as in the drawer of a nightstand or across the room with the clock face to the wall.

Relaxation Techniques

It is sometimes hard to determine the origin of your anxiety or lack of sleep. Over time, stressful situations can build up and cause feelings of helplessness or worry. The interrelated threads of stress, anxiety, sleep disruption, and insomnia pose an overwhelming challenge to your mental, emotional, and physical health. Consequently, I ask patients to incorporate relaxation into their daily schedule. Clear your schedule and your mind and kick anxiety and stress to the curb. Try these strategies for relaxation.

❯ Consider taking 1,000 units of vitamin E per day. Vitamin E is an excellent antioxidant that protects cellular membranes from a destructive process called lipid peroxidation. Free radicals looking for a negatively charged electron to achieve neutrality attach to electrons from lipids in the cell membrane, resulting in cellular damage.

❯ Increasing B vitamins during stress will help. B vitamins are used up and excreted in increasing amounts when under stress. The vitamins are necessary to form neurotransmitters such as serotonin and dopamine. B vitamins also prevent the buildup of

homocysteine, an inflammatory amino acid in the central nervous system, which may be the cause of anxiety and depression.

❯ In a journal, write quickly or deliberately slowly to focus all the thoughts going through your mind. Put the pen to paper and keep writing to control symptoms and diffuse tension.

❯ You can train yourself to tune out your surroundings by placing your right hand on your heart. The hand serves as a physical anchor to relax and let your tension fall away. Close your eyes to help deepen your focus.

❯ When your anxiety develops, get active in an exercise that requires your focus and energy.

❯ Take magnesium and vitamin C, which can be depleted during stress. Vitamin C serves as an antioxidant to produce the neurotransmitter norepinephrine from dopamine.

Any training that helps you relax, such as breathing exercises, biofeedback, yoga, guided imagery, and light hypnosis sleep tapes, are effective in getting you to sleep. You choose which activity you would enjoy, and that helps you feel quieter inside. These factors motivate you, so you don't feel like you have to work harder at sleeping.

If you have hyperarousal syndrome, an excessive responsiveness to sensory stimuli that causes causing you to overreact, several relaxation therapies help you retrain this anxiety pattern. I suggest patients undertake this type of intervention with support and guidance, or at least with an accountability partner. You must commit to a longer-term practice to establish new patterns in the brain and body, and being accountable to another person helps you stick to the protocol.

Entrain Your Circadian Rhythms

The parts of your brain and body regulating circadian rhythms take cues from your environment. Set parameters by following the steps below to regain internal balance and be in sync with your surroundings. This helps you feel in control again, your schedule becomes stabilized, and most of all, you are happier and sleep better.

Find a Consistent Sleep Cycle

Go to bed and get up at the same time each day to regulate your circadian rhythms. Eliminate the distraction of clock-watching so you can relax. Do not sleep later on weekends or nonwork days. The body's internal timer keeps getting confused when you do this. Keep a regular wake time seven days a week.

Do Not Linger in Bed

Spending excessive time in bed has three unfortunate consequences: (1) you begin to associate your bedroom with arousal and frustration, (2) your sleep becomes shallower and (3) you throw off your circadian sleep-wake schedule.

Use an alarm to set a definite schedule to wake up and get out of bed at the same time every morning, regardless of when you went to bed or how much you slept.

Go to Bed Only When You Are Sleepy

If you go to bed before you are sleepy, you have more time to become frustrated. Often people ponder the events of the day, review their task list, or worry about why they can't sleep. Therefore, delay your bedtime until you are sleepy, even if this means you go to bed later than your scheduled time.

Get Out of Bed When You Cannot Fall Asleep

Being in bed is for sleeping. The goal is for you to fall asleep quickly. If you cannot sleep, then get out of bed right away and go to another room to read, stretch, listen to music, or relax in the best way you can. When you feel sleepy again, return to bed. If you still cannot sleep, get out of bed and do something relaxing; do not work or be active on electronic devices. Return to bed only when you are sleepy. You are learning to associate your bed with sleeping rather than frustration. You are also more likely to go into deeper stages of sleep more quickly.

Use the Bedroom for Sleep Only

You might associate the kitchen with preparing, cooking, and eating foods. In the same way, you want to train your association of sleeping to your bedroom space and prevent negative feelings or worries about sleep. You may have to move the television, radio, or other electronic devices from your bedroom during this phase of sleep retraining.

Allow Yourself an Hour to Unwind Before Bedtime

Those who tend to worry or plan, or who are more active at night, have trouble switching off brain activity. This is not as easy as flipping a light switch. Take time to unwind. Take a hot bath or drink a hot cup of tea for relaxation. Don't do anything else that might increase your arousal. When you go to bed to sleep, aim to feel calm, peaceful, and relaxed.

> Use an alarm to set a definite schedule to wake up and get out of bed at the same time every morning, regardless of when you went to bed or how much you slept.

Retrain Your Sleep Patterns through Sleep Restriction Therapy

This program starts with you keeping a week's worth of sleep logs and calculating how much sleep you get as opposed to how long you lie in bed. This program recalibrates the internal clock by first permitting a minimum of five and a half hours of sleep or more per night, depending on how much sleep you calculate you actually get. Then you gradually increase the sleeping time by fifteen minutes each week when you can calculate that you slept at least 85 percent of the time you were in bed during the previous week. This method ensures the time spent in bed corresponds to the actual time you are sleeping, and not the total time spent trying to sleep. There is a significant difference between the two emotional states. Going to bed and trying to sleep is nerve-wracking and agitating. Going to bed to sleep when your body is sleepy is refreshing and restful. Here are three steps:

1. When you are in bed, you are there only to sleep. Limit the time in your bed not sleeping.

2. Go to sleep later, but maintain the same wake time.

3. Next, increase your time spent in bed by fifteen minutes per week. The goal is to show more than 85 percent sleep efficiency during the preceding week, according to your sleep expert's guidance, until you sleep all night.

Consider Hypnosis

Does hypnosis have a place in sleep medicine? A recent study showed the positive effects of hypnosis on sleep, especially deep sleep. Researchers enlisted seventy Swiss women, ages 18 to 35, and verified their malleability to hypnosis by the women's scores on the Harvard Group Scale of Hypnotic Susceptibility (HGSHS). The women listened to a 13-minute audiotape and were allowed to fall asleep for 90 minutes while listening or just after listening to the tape. During this time, researchers measured brain wave activity.

The findings were remarkable. Of the seventy women in the study, those who were suggestible to hypnosis and who listened to a tape full of metaphors for deep sleep, increased their deep sleep by 8 percent on average. Also, their time spent awake was reduced by 67 percent.

We know that deep sleep, or slow-wave sleep, decreases greatly with age. Also, commonly prescribed sleep medications, such as the benzodiazepines diazepam and temazepam, and

Sleep directly affects your ability to cope with and prevent infection.

the non-benzodiazepines such as zolpidem, diminish sleep. Such loss of deep sleep correlates directly with a decrease in cognitive function, deterioration in the immune system, impaired tissue repair, and age-related brain atrophy.

Hypnosis could have a place in treatment for insomnia for those susceptible to hypnotic therapy. Because this study showed an increase in deep sleep, it indicates that hypnosis could benefit the elderly population by preventing the usual deterioration of deep sleep seen with aging.

Try Tea and Tart Cherry Juice

Green tea contains L-theanine, an amino acid. One of its biological functions is to block the binding of L-glutamic acid (glutamate), which is the brain's main excitatory neurotransmitter. Without increasing drowsiness, L-theanine increases alpha brain wave levels.

Alpha brain waves are the slowest brain waves noted while awake, and they provide vividness and clarity to visualizations. Studies of brain waves, meditation, learning, and relaxation associate the alpha brain wave state with calmness and feelings of peace. You may notice that you go into an alpha state when you soak in a hot tub, relax in the shower, or daydream about that beach vacation. You should consider drinking a refreshing cup of green tea to promote alpha brain waves to calm anxiety and panic.

Chamomile tea is calming and supports sleep. It is proven to reduce anxiety, nightmares, and insomnia. One active ingredient called apigenin reduces locomotor activity, which disrupts sleep in restless sleepers. Also, the first controlled study of the use of chamomile extract showed that it has a moderate effect in reducing anxiety in people with general anxiety disorder.

Barley tea contains tryptophan, which is an amino acid necessary for sleep and helps you relax.

Siberian ginseng tea contains triterpenoid saponins, substances that reduce stress. This tea helps blood circulation and regulates the amount of stress you experience.

Tart cherry juice can help increase the amount of time you sleep. A recent study performed at Louisiana State University demonstrated that consuming two 8-ounce (235 ml) glasses of cherry juice a day increased sleep time by almost 90 minutes in older individuals. However, not just any cherry juice will do. Tart cherry juice works best because it contains melatonin, the sleep neurohormone, and also proanthocyanidin, which gives the juice that ruby color. Proanthocyanidin is an antioxidant that prevents the breakdown of tryptophan. Our bodies convert the amino acid tryptophan into the serotonin and melatonin needed for sleeping. A variation of the drink is to make a smoothie at night by adding frozen tart cherries to almond milk or coconut milk. I also add a little yogurt, banana, and cinnamon for a distinctive flavor.

These rituals truly allow time for you to care for you: finish chores, feel relaxed, quiet your mind, and release your worries and burdens of the day.

Get Your Vitamins

Vitamin D deficiency is linked to hypersomnia, a condition where you are overly sleepy throughout the day. It also has been linked to restless legs syndrome, which can keep you from falling asleep or staying asleep. (See more on restless legs syndrome on page 118.) Vitamin D also maintains the brain's neurotransmitters, and deficiencies have been linked to increased insomnia in the elderly and to muscle aches and pains that disturb sleep. The best way to get enough vitamin D is exposure to sunlight. You can also take vitamin D supplements. If you can get direct sunlight exposure after waking, you will start your day well. If you suffer from any of the above symptoms, ask your health-care provider to check your vitamin D levels. (See chapter 9 for more on nutrient-dense food.)

Sleep Habits to Avoid

Your activities during the day influence how well you sleep at night. How much physical activity do you get? If you are mostly sedentary, the lack of physical activity can be affecting your sleep. How mentally stimulated are you during daytime and nighttime activities? If you have trouble turning off mentally or putting work or focused mental activities aside at least one hour before sleeping, you could be setting

TO DO:
ELIMINATE THESE STIMULANTS

The following are stimulants that interfere with sleep and should be reduced or avoided entirely.

① **Alcohol**

② **Caffeine** (including chocolate and caffeinated beverages) If you consume caffeine, stop at least six hours before sleeping, or remove it from your diet completely, especially if you are over sixty-five years of age.

③ **Cigarettes**

Also, talk to your health-care provider about any medications you take that may contribute to or cause insomnia. Do not stop or adjust any medications without your physician's advice.

yourself up for insomnia. Here are some other habits to avoid.

Pets

Do not sleep with pets unless they contribute significantly to your sleep. Do not undermine your health because of what you feel your cat or dog may want, need, or demand. Sleeping without a pet may be a tough habit to break. However, you are riding

TO DO:

ELIMINATE THESE DISTRACTIONS

It's important that you associate your bed and bedroom with sleep and not other activities that can interfere with sleep. Eliminating these distractions will make your bedroom a more restful place.

① Reading in bed

② Watching television in the bedroom

③ Using electronic devices (including the phone, tablet, or computer) in bed

④ Allowing pets in bed or the bedroom

⑤ Eating while in bed

the change for them as much as for yourself: You will be a much better caretaker if you are well rested.

Nicotine

Using nicotine before bed is counterproductive. After the first puff from a cigarette, nicotine promotes the release of the brain neurotransmitter acetylcholine. This powerful chemical increases the activity of the brain's reticular activating system, the brain's wake-promoting circuit.

Alcohol

Alcohol initially induces sleep and promotes increased deep sleep. That marks the end of any benefit, as your body metabolizes the alcohol and provokes withdrawal. That triggers an increase in stress hormones such as adrenaline and noradrenaline and a rebound of wakefulness. Once awake, you will likely struggle to return to sleep.

Sleep and alcohol use are firmly entangled because many people have a nightcap before going to bed. Yet, insomnia is the greatest predictor for alcoholic relapses. Those who enjoy a nightcap think it will help them fall asleep, but it does not help them achieve good-quality sleep or enough sleep.

Initially, alcohol acts on areas of the brain in the same way that sleeping pills affect the brain. An alcoholic drink enhances deep sleep and suppresses REM (dream) sleep in the first half of the night. However, as the body metabolizes the alcohol, body temperature increases and stress hormones are released, resulting in frequent arousals, difficulty remaining asleep, and a marked increase in the second half of the night in REM sleep, bringing on vivid and disturbing dreams. Alcohol also suppresses the hypothalamus's ability to decrease the production of cortisol when hormone levels rise. The result is just the opposite of your intended goal to sleep well for seven to nine hours. Instead, the switch that moderates cortisol turns off, and the body continues to produce elevated concentrations of cortisol. Within a week, the person drinking nightcaps will feel the need for more alcohol to get to sleep.

Even if a person abstained from alcohol, sleep abnormalities in former alcohol users can persist for up to two years. Such an extended inhibition of REM sleep increases the amount of REM sleep called REM rebound. The results could include frequent nightmares and disturbing dreams, which often make the person start drinking again.

Alcohol also poses other serious problems in those with sleep apnea. Alcohol relaxes the upper airway muscles, causing a more severe collapse than might normally occur, and weakens the brain's ability to respond effectively to the obstruction. This kind of preventable health issue is a more dangerous situation for people who have untreated sleep apnea.

To get good quality, uninterrupted sleep, remember these points:

⟩ Never use alcohol as a sleep aid.
⟩ If you are a recovering alcoholic with sleep problems, address the issue immediately with your physician.
⟩ Alcohol use worsens sleep disorders such as sleep apnea and nightmare disturbances.

⟩ Alcohol causes an overproduction of cortisol that exacerbates further inflammation and deregulates the immune system.
⟩ Alcohol disrupts the formation of new brain cells, especially in the cerebellum area associated with motor function.
⟩ Alcohol can make the brain's receptors less sensitive to neurotransmitters such as serotonin, dopamine, and norepinephrine, and this may contribute to why so many alcoholics suffer from associated depression and anxiety.

Stimulants

Caffeine contributes to insomnia because metabolizing caffeine can take from four to ten hours and is dependent on an individual's metabolism. I suggest eliminating caffeine, or at least curtailing caffeine intake after 10 a.m. If you have severe headaches when limiting caffeine products, I recommend a 50 percent reduction every two days until you are off caffeine.

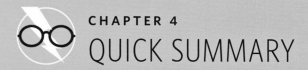

CHAPTER 4
QUICK SUMMARY

⟩ You get healthier sleep at night when stimulants do not contribute to arousal and wakefulness.

⟩ Likewise, distracting behaviors that also stimulate your thoughts can become habits that keep you awake.

⟩ Sleep hygiene and bedtime preparation enable you to tailor your sleep environment to your needs.

⟩ Establishing relaxation rituals helps diminish stress and creates a consistent sleep cycle.

⟩ Irritability, moodiness, fatigue, fuzzy thinking, and headaches also result from lost sleep.

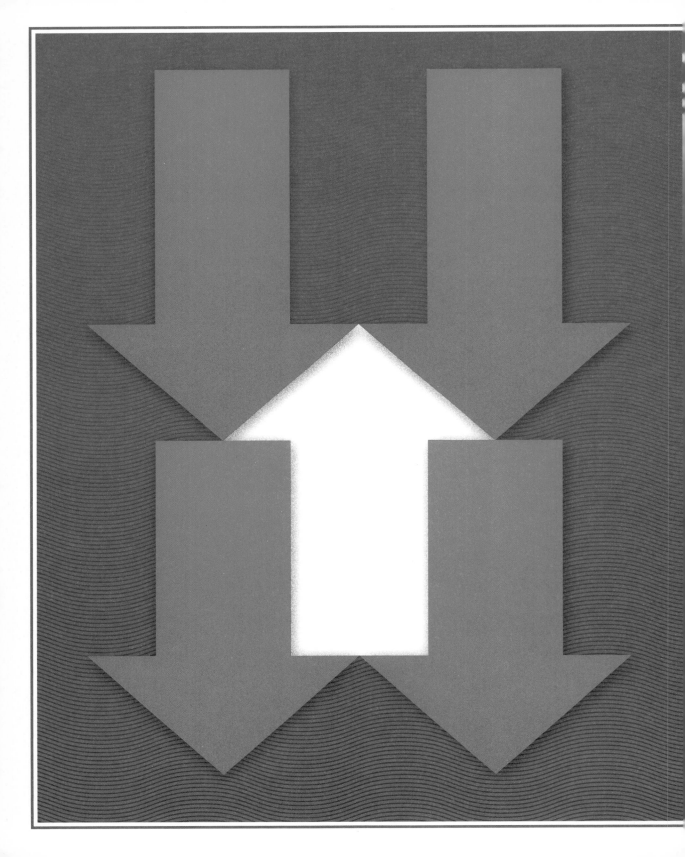

CHAPTER 5

THE PHYSIOLOGICAL EFFECTS OF STRESS AND HOW WE ADAPT

In simplest terms, stress is the body's response to a stimulus that interferes with normal physiology and functioning. Being stressed means feeling out of balance.

Bring to mind a difficult situation or condition you have recently faced. When you consider how you responded, did you feel drained emotionally, mentally, or physically? You experience stress when you perceive that the demands on your energy exceed your supply of energy.

Bodies have natural reserves of energy that are vital to your health. You need energy as part of your life support system, as necessary as respiration and circulation. There are different types of stress. How you perceive stress influences how the distress or eustress affects you mentally, emotionally, and physically.

Another way to look at distress is how it disrupts the process of homeostasis, which is the body in proper balance with regard to temperature, electrolyte concentrations, and acid-base. Allostasis is the active process through which your body responds to stress in an attempt to maintain homeostasis (balance). However, when stress is chronic, you develop what is called

an *allosteric load*, the wear and tear on the body from chronic stress, as the body attempts to maintain balance or equilibrium.

Stress Response in the Body

To best understand how stress occurs and affects the body, consider the following example.

Jenna and Frank are the proud parents of three-year-old twins. They were glad to be over the infant and toddler years, feeling as though they rarely slept because they devoted every minute to the twins.

Jenna recently found out that she was pregnant again. Her altruistic heart would always welcome another child. However, her thoughts were filled with worry and self-doubt. She couldn't discuss it with anyone, because everyone around her was excited about the possibility of a younger sister for the twin boys. Jenna hid her reservations during the day around family and friends. However, at night, when no one could guess at her doubts and fears, she worried and found it increasingly more difficult to fall and stay asleep. Then she woke up tired and moody. The twins were too young to know why

Threat System (Fight or Flight)

A stress response activates a fight-or-flight process
in the sympathetic nervous system.

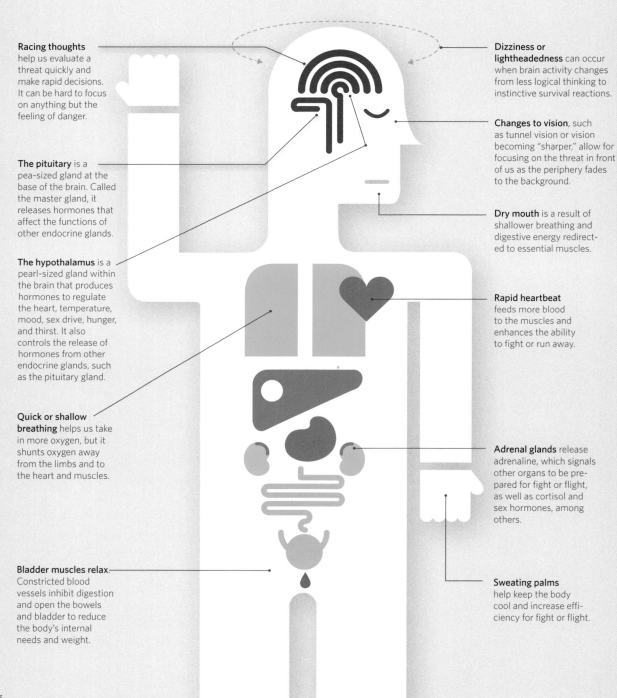

Racing thoughts
help us evaluate a
threat quickly and
make rapid decisions.
It can be hard to focus
on anything but the
feeling of danger.

The pituitary is a
pea-sized gland at the
base of the brain. Called
the master gland, it
releases hormones that
affect the functions of
other endocrine glands.

The hypothalamus is a
pearl-sized gland within
the brain that produces
hormones to regulate
the heart, temperature,
mood, sex drive, hunger,
and thirst. It also
controls the release of
hormones from other
endocrine glands, such
as the pituitary gland.

**Quick or shallow
breathing** helps us take
in more oxygen, but it
shunts oxygen away
from the limbs and to
the heart and muscles.

Bladder muscles relax.
Constricted blood
vessels inhibit digestion
and open the bowels
and bladder to reduce
the body's internal
needs and weight.

**Dizziness or
lightheadedness** can occur
when brain activity changes
from less logical thinking to
instinctive survival reactions.

Changes to vision, such
as tunnel vision or vision
becoming "sharper," allow
for focusing on the threat in front
of us as the periphery fades
to the background.

Dry mouth is a result of
shallower breathing and
digestive energy redirect-
ed to essential muscles.

Rapid heartbeat
feeds more blood
to the muscles and
enhances the ability
to fight or run away.

Adrenal glands release
adrenaline, which signals
other organs to be pre-
pared for fight or flight,
as well as cortisol and
sex hormones, among
others.

Sweating palms
help keep the body
cool and increase effi-
ciency for fight or flight.

mom was irritable and lying about being happy. She worried, too, about her ability to be a good mother to three children under four years of age. Jenna's stress reactions and the results of her worry follow the patterns that you might recognize.

From the perspective of evolution, the stress response has evolved as an important defensive tool for adaptation. We call it the fight-flight-freeze response. The amygdala filters sensory information. If it perceives a threat, the amygdala notifies the hypothalamus, which serves as a command center. Next, the sympathetic nervous system activates the fight-or-flight response.

Jenna's continued worries about the pregnancy and her moodiness shows the HPA axis at work. It controls reactions to stress and trauma and maintains alertness. Dysfunction of the HPA axis at any level also disrupts sleep. The hypothalamus releases a hormone called corticotropin-releasing hormone (CRH), which in turn stimulates the pituitary gland to release adrenocorticotropic hormone (ACTH). Then the adrenals secrete cortisol and other hormones that send chemical messages: "All systems go. Mobilize the forces. Danger lurks." Danger could be a hungry grizzly bear or the slow driver you are trying to pass in heavy traffic. In Jenna's case, her continued fearful perceptions kept her system alert, awake, and worrying about danger.

At the same time, the hypothalamus triggered her sympathetic nervous system to release the stress hormones noradrenaline and adrenaline. After such adrenaline rushes, one choice Jenna had was to relax and not feel threatened by her pregnancy. However, Jenna's HPA system remained elevated, which increased production of

TERM REVIEW

Stress refers to mental, emotional, environmental, or physical factors causing tension in your body or mind.

Eustress refers to happy, fulfilling, or pleasurable experiences and contributes more energy to your bank. Good stress stretches you a little and helps you achieve your goals.

Distress refers to taxing, painful, insulting, or tiring experiences that drain energy from your bank. Distress interferes with your physiology.

Stressors cause stress reactions. They are conditions or situations that make demands on your energy.

Acute stress refers to the rapid onset of stress of short duration.

Chronic stress refers to persistent, longer term, frequently recurring, or longer lasting stress.

cortisol and resulted in exhaustion. If her hyper-arousal continued throughout her pregnancy, the HPA would determine this state to be Jenna's new normal. This would force a lower set point for her stress threshold, allowing stress to occur more easily. Chronic elevations of cortisol decrease our brain's response to important neurotransmitters such as dopamine, serotonin, and norepinephrine.

We need these hormones to regulate mood and modulate reactions to stress. Thus, she became increasingly sensitive to her environment, making her more prone to stress responses.

Adaptation

How well you adapt to situations is essential to your well-being. Some people adapt internally by changing their attitudes, thoughts, or feelings about a situation. Sometimes you can take charge of the environment or situation and feel in control again. Such coping skills involve what you think, how you feel, your energy levels, and your perceptions.

What you *think* while under stress can help you adapt or work counter to your efforts. For example, when Jenna found out about her second pregnancy, her mind filled with worry and likely some guilt for having doubts. After accepting her pregnancy, other odd thoughts also filled her mind: Would her husband still support her? Would her friends judge her if she admitted her doubts? Why did her mother need to nag her about a granddaughter? Unhelpful thinking worsened when she grew apprehensive about the worries she had. Her nighttime worry escalated to anxiety that kept her awake and agitated. Basically, she had developed a cascade of negative and automatic thoughts. By automatic we mean that they occur quickly, are uninvited, seem plausible, and make you feel worse.

What you *feel*—in other words, your emotional state—can activate and escalate stress. Jenna always saw herself as a mild-mannered, average woman and joked that Supermom could handle twin boys by herself. Now she felt stupid that she had bragged about being Supermom. Her emotional state ranged from irritability during the day to anxiety and worry at night. Moreover, she withdrew from others for fear of showing weakness.

Your brain and body react and show symptoms when distressed. Do you pay attention to those symptoms? Do you push through, persevere, freeze, cry, withdraw, take charge, or ask for support? For Jenna, she could not seem to turn off her worry. Her restless thoughts extended from the night jitters into daytime apprehensions. She was weary and cried more often. She was afraid to ask for help.

CHECK-IN:
IDENTIFY SIGNS OF DISTRESS

Review the following signs of distress and check the ones you experience.

Physical
- ◯ Tension headaches
- ◯ Nausea
- ◯ Sweating
- ◯ Indigestion
- ◯ Skin breaks out
- ◯ Agitation
- ◯ Tiredness and sleep disturbance

Behavioral
- ◯ Changes in appetite
- ◯ Avoidance
- ◯ Low productivity
- ◯ Impatience
- ◯ Rush to action
- ◯ Change in sleeping patterns

Cognitive
- ◯ Poor decision making
- ◯ Exaggerated responses
- ◯ Carelessness
- ◯ Overly sensitive
- ◯ Muddled thinking
- ◯ Feelings of fear and dread
- ◯ Defensive
- ◯ Constant worry/anxiety

Emotional
- ◯ Mood swings
- ◯ Feelings of guilt
- ◯ Withdrawal
- ◯ Lack of sense of humor
- ◯ Feelings of being alone

A study of 3,000 participants found that people who encountered stressors more frequently or had more exposure to stressors were more likely to experience insomnia.

How you manage or cope when under distress also affects your *energy levels*. Jenna knew better than to hide her feelings of being overwhelmed or sad. However, she felt blocked and could not speak up or get help, and she was exhausted all the time. She denied her moodiness when her husband or mother asked her how she was holding up.

Finally, your *perceptions* influence your responses to stress and ability to manage stress overloads. Jenna perceived her situation as negative and overwhelming. Her thoughts about the pregnancy included worries and fears. Her emotional states ranged from irritability to worrying to feeling afraid. Her behavior included withdrawing from friends and family, not sharing much, and not asking for help or emotional support. The results were disrupted sleep, lack of energy, and emotional overreactivity. Chapter 6 examines the role of perceptions on stress.

Jenna finally recognized that her sleep deficiency made her emotions worse. Lack of sleep itself is a major stressor. She came to the sleep clinic to learn healthier coping skills so she could sleep better. I explained to Jenna that HPA activation meant that she had been on high alert for a while and her brain and body stayed awake and alert to danger.

We started a program of cognitive behavioral therapy. Jenna went to bed only when sleepy and got out of bed if wide awake after twenty minutes and practiced a calming activity.

We also began a program of cognitive restructuring. Jenna wrote down these automatic negative thoughts, challenged them, and replaced them with more positive and truthful cognitions. She did this upon waking in the morning while they were fresh in her mind and again in the early evening.

Finally, Jenna kept daily sleep diaries. By the second week, she was beginning to see a change in her sleep. Where it used to take her ninety minutes to fall asleep, it eventually reduced to thirty minutes. Her time awake after falling asleep decreased from two hours to forty-five minutes. She continued the program during her pregnancy and by the sixth week, she was sleeping a solid six and a half to seven and a half hours a night.

When Distress Escalates

When you go to sleep, the HPA axis is suppressed. In the early morning hours before you awaken, your body increases secretion of cortisol. Cortisol peaks and is highest at about thirty minutes after we awaken and is referred to as the cortisol awakening response (CAR). However, escalating stress disrupts the normal circadian rhythms of the HPA axis and causes nocturnal elevation of cortisol, which disrupts sleep.

Emotional reactivity appears as a high startle response, increased sensitivity to pain, excessive worry, anxiety, and fatigue. It also causes inflammation, which at first is protective and appropriate, but with chronicity, it becomes damaging. Elevated cortisol and other stress hormones also disrupt eating schedules, mood regulation, and emotionality. The HPA axis is activated and disrupts sleep. The result is insomnia that triggers more fears or worries about not being able to sleep.

How you evaluate and then cope with stress may increase your risk of insomnia. Researchers from Henry Ford Hospital were the first to study how cognitive intrusions such as worry or ruminations affect sleep. The study of 3,000 participants found that people who encountered stressors more frequently or had more exposure to stressors were more likely to experience insomnia. The cognitive intrusions that disrupted normal thinking also increased. A stressful event can lead to a night of little sleep. However, your stress response and perception are the difference between one bad night of sleep and developing insomnia. In this study, the three coping behaviors that served as mediators were behavioral disengagement, distraction, and substance use.

Behavioral disengagement refers to giving up on the stress, the equivalent of throwing in the towel. Distraction is about focusing your attention elsewhere instead of managing stress.

Substance abuse is another diversion tactic, which might help one cope in the short term but may only exacerbate the root issue. Before troublesome thoughts escalate to rumination, and worry escalates to anxiety, recognize these symptoms as a possible state of hyperarousal. Your health depends on your ability to be aware if you experience stress that expands and continues for prolonged periods.

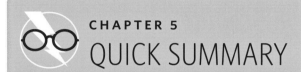

CHAPTER 5

QUICK SUMMARY

Recognize the different types of stress responses. Is your response to stress a healthy one?

» **Positive:** Short bursts of stress increase stress hormones and heart rate. Stress is intermittent.

» **Reasonable:** Serious temporary stress overload is buffered in some way by its short duration, a one-time event, supportive relationships, or other aspects that cushion the impact.

» **Toxic:** Stress responses are overwhelming, persistent, or prolonged and could include the absence of supportive help or buffers.

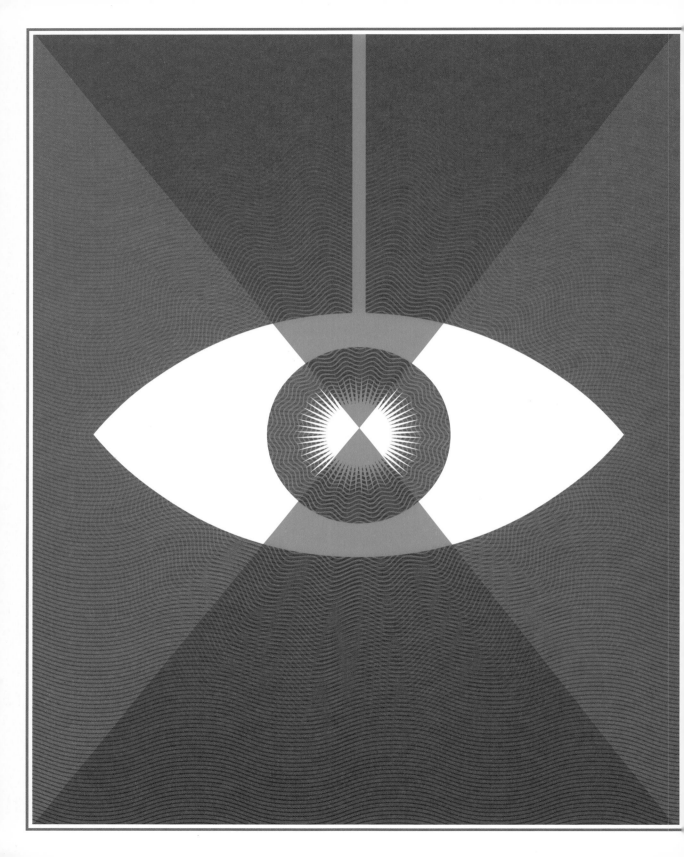

CHAPTER 6

HOW THE BRAIN PROCESSES FEAR AND HOW YOU PERCEIVE STRESS

How you respond to distressing events highly influences how you feel and how resilient you can be. Jenna's case, explored in the previous chapter, demonstrates a person who internalizes her feelings and copes with problems negatively and emotionally when stressed, which triggers the HPA cascade of cortisol. Prolonged elevated cortisol disrupts memory by shrinking the hippocampus. It also causes neuroreceptors to be less responsive to neurotransmitters, such as serotonin, dopamine, and norepinephrine, which are what you need to improve mood, alertness, and anxiety. Most important are the structural alterations in the amygdala from a continuous cortisol cascade.

The Role of the Amygdala

For its small size, the amygdala packs a lot of power to influence emotions and emotional behavior. Overall, the amygdala is responsible for perceptions of threat, control of aggression, and control of the responses that help you deal with a threat.

The amygdala is actually two small, almond-shaped groups of nuclei; each amygdala is located within each temporal lobe and has a specified function in processing emotional information. The right-hemisphere amygdala functions are associated with handling fear-related stimuli and negative emotions and influences the expression of fear. The right amygdala also has a role in associating time and place to emotions. The left-hemisphere amygdala functions are associated with handling pleasant sensations, such as happiness. Researchers theorize that the left-hemisphere amygdala is part of the brain's reward system.

Over the years, neuroscientists have mapped the amygdala's role in mental states and disorders. In children with anxiety disorders, the amygdala is smaller than normal. The use of antidepressant medications as well as psychotherapy can increase the size of the amygdala.

Links between the Amygdala and Anxiety and Panic

More women than men experience anxiety and are more affected than men are to that anxiety. The amygdala can trigger anxiety and panic attacks when it senses environmental threats, but

Fear, stress, and anxiety are not based in circumstances, but in perspective.

what kicks the amygdala into action? In addition to visually sensing a threat, other triggers could include smells, emotions, tastes, sounds, or pain. The amygdala processes almost all external sensory inputs, called the unconditional stimulus (UCS), in part due to past encounters, which are stored memories that trigger the autonomic nervous system and the HPA axis responses.

The Amygdala's Role in Sleep

Lack of sleep is common in people who experience anxiety, worry, and rumination. Lack of sleep also ramps up the amygdala, the insular cortex, and subsequently negative emotions, because this area of the brain contributes to emotional processing. Research has verified that any lack of sleep means your brain and body cannot repair and renew neurobiological systems. Sleep therapy offers a very real, possible treatment for symptoms of distress, anxiety, and panic, as well as psychiatric disorders that may develop from these conditions. We've known for decades that sleep disturbances and mental health disorders occur together. Now this recent research has shown there is a causal relationship: Sleep loss triggers a large amount of anticipatory brain behavior—that is, expected reactions that are associated with anxiety.

How the Amygdala Hijacks the Rational Brain

The hippocampus is the learning center in the brain that converts new information into long-term memory storage. Every night as you sleep, this region of the brain in the temporal lobe uploads the day's learning experiences into the higher cortical centers. There, consolidation of learning experiences and sensory input occur through neuron production and laying out new pathways. Acute stress or prolonged exposure to disastrous events releases stress hormones. Cortisol then attacks the hippocampus by reducing neurons and shrinking it.

When emotion meets memory, the amygdala and hippocampus are communicating. The hippocampus signals the amygdala, which processes new information that is fearful or threatening. The amygdala activates the HPA axis, the sympathetic nervous system, and then hijacks the rational brain. Connections to the prefrontal cortex, where executive function comes from, are decreased. The amygdala's fear prompts are good for survival but not so good for anxiety behavior. The hippocampus and the amygdala rely on each other for the right signals to function properly.

Fostering Resilience

The human system is as resilient as it is sensitive. Just as an earthquake can shrink the hippocampus

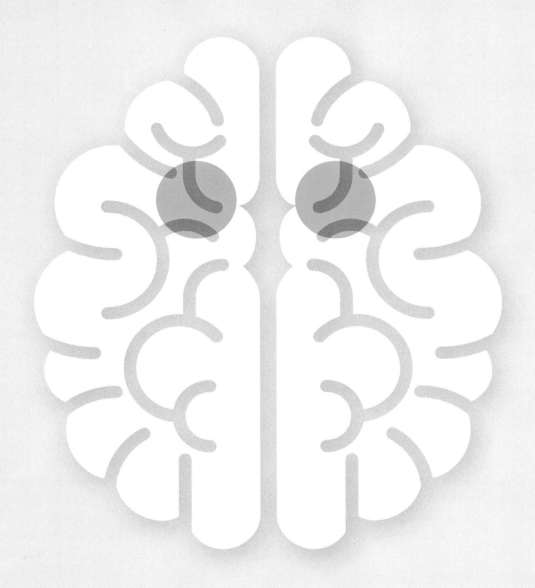

The Amygdala(e)

What we generally call the amygdala is actually two separate amygdalae, or groups of nuclei. Each amygdala processes different types of emotional information.

and consolidate fear memories in survivors, certain therapies can heal fearful memories. Medications can assist in blocking those fear memories. Sleep can restore and repair.

Within the amygdala, certain proteins are required to consolidate fear memories. If a medication disrupts this protein creation process, then fearful, conditioned responses are not stored as memories. One such drug inhibitor is UO 126, and when it was delivered within the amygdala of rats conditioned to fear, the rats' brains forgot the fear responses.

During sleep, the amygdala and hippocampus communicate with the prefrontal cortex, and negative emotions change through fear extinction. Extinction is a process in which we replace the fear-triggering association with one that does not trigger negative emotional and physiological reactions. Specific therapies can accomplish this task. In exposure therapy, for example, a therapist asks you to recount and visualize the anxiety-provoking trigger. By doing so, you develop more positive associations that replace the provoking trigger. You need healthy sleep for any therapies used in anxiety treatments and PTSD treatments to be successful because this process

seems to be especially dependent on REM sleep. Remember, insufficient sleep due to stress and anxiety inhibits and obstructs the process of erasing fears, making it impossible to control fear and anxiety. For this reason, you must get good sleep while undergoing therapy to solidify the positive associations.

Traumatic Life Events and Resilience

The ways in which stressful events affect you personally depends on how you interpret the event or what you believe about it. For one person, a divorce could be liberating. For another, divorce could be devastating.

To find out more about divorce and its effects on stress, researchers studied 138 individuals in the process of separation or divorce. The participants reported their sleep complaints and had their blood pressure taken in a laboratory three times during the nearly eight months of monitoring. Researchers found that sleep complaints predicted significant increases in blood pressure at follow-up visits. Sleep problems during the first ten weeks post-separation were not associated with persistent increases in blood pressure, but those with persistent sleep problems after ten weeks experienced chronic elevations in blood pressure.

This study is not the first one to highlight the relationship between divorce, sleep, and blood pressure elevation, a stress marker. A 2009 study came to a similar conclusion that divorce-related, emotional difficulty played a significant role in elevating blood pressure, particularly in men.

Everyone experiences stress, but how stress affects you depends on your perceptions. A remarkable British cohort study shows this connection. The researchers followed 7,268 men and women whose average age was 49.5 years for eighteen years. People reported whether stress affected their health at the start of the study. Those who reported that stress did affect their health had a 2.5 times greater risk for a coronary event than those who reported that stress had no effect on their health.

Traumatic, large-scale events, such as earthquakes, give researchers another opportunity to study how stress affects a large number of people. We know that those who experience a major upheaval or loss are at greater risk of sudden death. For example, studies found a correlated link between those who experienced a major earthquake in Los Angeles in 1994 and the increased number of people who died from sudden heart attacks. Social scientists studied similar heart health statistics before and after the terrorist attacks on September 11, 2001, in two groups of people in New Haven, Connecticut. The post-9/11 group showed lower heart-rate variability, a marker of an overactive sympathetic nervous system, which is a high-risk factor for sudden death.

A study about the long-term effects of the September 11, 2001, attacks and similar events has shown how people exhibited one of three coping patterns. Those with poor coping skills suffered from intrusive memories, chronic distress, or longer term sorrow. The middle group had intense reactions but eventually managed to function as they had before the event. The third group displayed the best coping skills, with reactions of shorter duration, fewer than anticipated repercussions, and remarkable resilience. This group returned to healthy functioning more quickly than the others.

Resilience and the Brain

Why do some people cope much better than others do when larger-than-life events cause suffering and loss, even though such events impact the affected population in similar ways? We know that some people can and do adjust quickly after absorbing the initial impact of a traumatic event. Studies suggest that your recovery might directly connect to how you think of yourself. Self-esteem played a significant role in how survivors of the 2011 earthquake in Japan recovered emotionally. Researchers conducted brain scans after the quake to compare with brain scans conducted before the earthquake to see how the stress of the earthquake affected people's brains. The researchers noted that, after disasters, alterations in the brain endured for years afterward. The regions of the brain that were diminished after the earthquake were the orbitofrontal cortex and the hippocampus.

The orbitofrontal cortex is highly sensitive to the detrimental effects of stress exposure as well as sleep deprivation. Prolonged exposure deregulates stress-signaling systems. The result is a loss of emotional control and clear judgment. Acute stress or prolonged exposure to disastrous events releases stress hormones, including cortisol, which attacks the hippocampus by reducing neurons and shrinking it.

The Japan study continued for twelve months after the earthquake and showed the hippocampus still shrinking in the individuals monitored who still had high stress. However, survivors who had healthier self-esteem and who did not experience significant sleep loss or nightmares after the trauma showed growth in the orbitofrontal region. Researchers believe the tissue regrowth was linked directly to the earthquake survivors' ability to cope and regulate their emotionality.

How do brain changes and long-term stress affect sleep patterns? Other researchers in Japan evaluated the sleep habits of 1,919 junior high school students at eight months and twenty months after the earthquake. One consistent finding was that children in the disaster regions had a decrease in sleep duration at eight months and also at twenty months, especially during weekdays. These children also continued to have trouble falling sleep and exhibited symptoms of insomnia and disrupted circadian rhythms at twenty months.

These findings show that acute events or prolonged exposure to stress creates a neurological problem, in addition to a psychological one, which disrupts the sleep-wake cycle. However, a strong sense of self-esteem helps people get through traumatic events. This is another excellent reason to participate in stress-relieving exercises that strengthen resilience and self-esteem. (Read more about improving self-esteem in chapter 8.) Healthy sleep after a traumatic event also plays a significant role in survivors' coping mechanisms. The brain and body need the process of fear extinction memory that occurs while sleeping. And we know that to be resilient to stress we must (1) change our perceptions about stress being bad or good, and (2) know that even if we have no control over a situation, we do have control over our emotional reactions and perceptions.

The Vicious Cycle

We now know that psychological stress triggers a reaction by the HPA and sympathetic nervous system. Moreover, it also sets off a cascade of inflammatory cytokines and destructive oxidative stress. The inflammatory cycle causes damage to nerves and receptors where neurotransmitters such as serotonin, norepinephrine, and dopamine affect mood, memory, and emotional processing. The result is sobering. Your ability to deal with stress deteriorates, sending you into a downward spiral. Lack of sleep only intensifies and worsens these changes. Sleep disturbances add to the inflammatory burden that overwhelms your ability to maintain physiological and psychological balance.

The best way to live well, sleep well, and remain in good health is to understand your vulnerabilities and how you perceive them. Do you believe that stress has a negative impact on your health? Or do you think that you have some level of control over the stressful events in your life? If you lose control of what is happening, how resilient are you in recovery or healing? Next, identify your strengths and how you can build personal resilience and healthy sleep hygiene. Know that you have tools to help you, and you should not hesitate to seek professional help after trauma.

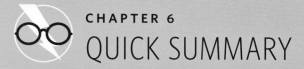

CHAPTER 6

QUICK SUMMARY

- Traumatic events affect the hippocampus and the orbitofrontal cortex.

- In addition to neurological problems, prolonged stress disrupts the sleep-wake cycle.

- How resilient a person is in coping with acute events or prolonged stress depends on self-esteem and the ability to sleep to allow neurobiological repairs.

- Healthy self-esteem—that is, having self-respect and personal values—increases one's ability to recover more quickly from acute events.

- Good sleep hygiene helps one sleep better and builds resilience.

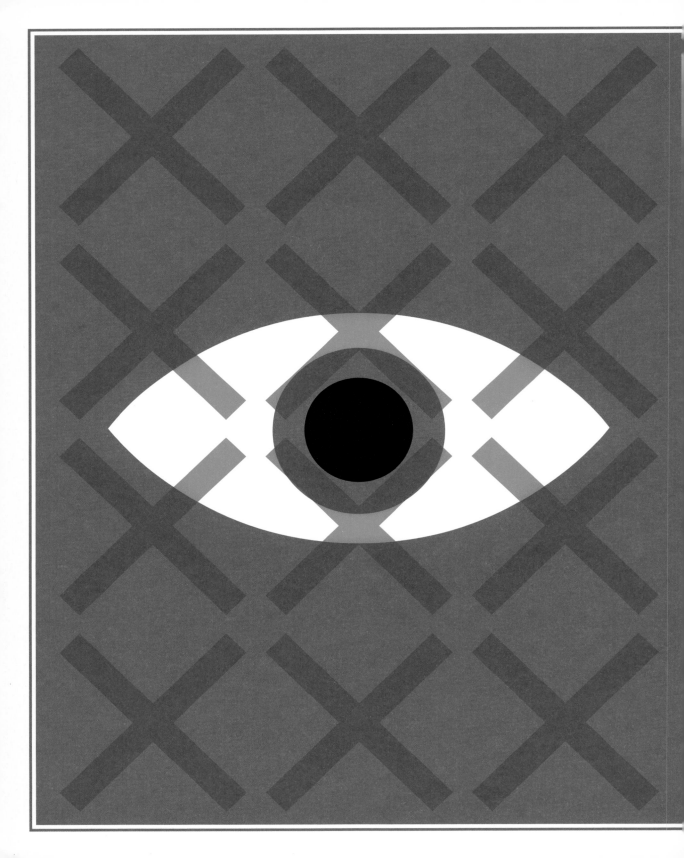

CHAPTER 7

INSOMNIA TYPES AND TREATMENTS

Who is most prone to insomnia? After a stressful event, many people experience transient insomnia that lasts for a short period. But those most vulnerable to stress-induced insomnia have poor coping skills. They ruminate and worry more, especially around bedtime. They have an overactive sympathetic (fight-or-flight) nervous system, a hyperactive HPA axis, and hyperarousal from an overproduction of stress hormones. This predisposes them to a more chronic form of insomnia.

Those who come to sleep specialists with the usual complaint of "I can't shut my mind down"; i.e., it is difficult for them to fall or stay asleep, often suffering from intrusive thoughts, also called cognitive intrusions or automatic negative thoughts.

Causes of Insomnia

Although there are various causes for insomnia, the two prevailing theories cite a physical and a psychological cause.

One reason you may have insomnia is the hyperarousal theory, where the brain and body stay in an alert, conscious state. When insomniacs are asleep, there is faster and more brain wave activity. Insomniacs' brains during sleep appear to be more active than those of normal sleepers. This is reflected by the appearance of faster brain waves and increased uptake of glucose, both of which are characteristic of wakefulness. This could be a primary reason that 50 percent of insomniacs severely underestimate their actual time asleep. Their brains are more active during sleep and they have more difficulty falling and staying asleep.

The second reason people have insomnia is the psychological theory. Insomnia sufferers seem to have anxiety-prone personalities and may be ruminators and worriers. They tend to exhibit poor coping skills, relying on emotions, and internalize their emotions. Their responses are highly reactive to chronic daily stressors.

One treatment does not fit all people with insomnia. Sleep experts sometimes need to combine pharmacologic treatment with cognitive behavioral therapy for insomnia, even if for a short period, to achieve the goal of getting quality sleep.

No matter what your age or gender, insomnia can happen to you. The following is a list of inherent traits and life stressors that could increase your vulnerability to insomnia:

- ⟩ Hyperarousal (chronic state of alert)
- ⟩ Family history of insomnia
- ⟩ Tendency to worry
- ⟩ Anxiety-prone personality
- ⟩ Preoccupation with well-being
- ⟩ Dramatic responsiveness to life events
- ⟩ Environmental factors such as living near traffic noise

In sleep medicine, we diagnose insomnia by gathering several types of information. General questions include any conditions that would keep you from sleeping well: Do you have any psychological condition or issue? Has a doctor diagnosed you with anxiety, depression, or other condition? You'll be queried regarding snoring and any current weight gain that might indicate a form of sleep apnea.

We also investigate sleep habits and other contributing factors through a sleep diary with entries for at least two weeks and other assessments. The inventories could include the Epworth Sleepiness Scale and the General Anxiety Disorder Scale.

How you deal with insomnia most often perpetuates the insomnia for several reasons. You may have persistent stressors such as illness, work schedule changes, lack of healthy sleep, or interpersonal conflicts that enhance your stress reactions and contribute to insomnia. Chronic stress results in a state of hyperarousal. Researchers presenting an overview of chronic insomnia and stress also labeled it as not so much a state of losing sleep as a hyperarousal disorder that is consistent throughout the day and night.

Recent evidence indicates that those with insomnia show hyperarousal of the central nervous system and disrupted sleep. If you experience a state of hyperarousal and are at risk for insomnia, a sleep doctor may see the following:

- ⟩ Electroencephalography (EEG), which records electrical brain activity, showing less slow-wave sleep and periods of rather rapid activity called beta during sleep
- ⟩ The activated sympathetic nervous system in a state of the fight-or-flight response
- ⟩ Lower than normal levels of melatonin and growth hormone, and higher levels of cortisol and adrenaline

TERM REVIEW

Insomnia means difficulty in getting to sleep and staying asleep, and waking earlier than normal.

The phrase **short-term insomnia** applies when insomnia symptoms have existed for fewer than three months and may be related to a stressor that is temporary or signifigant.

The term **chronic insomnia** occurs at least three times a week for a period of three or more months. Research in the last five years has made clear that insomnia is a chronic disease associated with arousal.

TO DO:
INSOMNIA SEVERITY INDEX

Difficulty getting to sleep and staying asleep are insomnia symptoms. Take the Insomnia Severity Index (ISI) and determine your sleeping pattern. You will learn whether your sleep issue is mild, moderate, or severe. This index provides a rating scale from 0 (no problem) to 4 (very severe) for each sleep problem. For every problem, rate the severity *only* for the past two weeks. Circle the number that best describes your answer.

Insomnia Severity Index

Insomnia problem	None	Mild	Moderate	Severe	Very severe
① Do you have difficulty falling asleep?	⓪	①	②	③	④
② Do you have difficulty staying asleep?	⓪	①	②	③	④
③ Do you wake up too early?	⓪	①	②	③	④
④ How **satisfied/dissatisfied** are you with your current sleep pattern?	⓪ Very satisfied	① Satisfied	② Moderately satisfied	③ Dissatisfied	③ Dissatisfied
⑤ How **noticeable** to others do you think your sleep problem is in terms of impairing the quality of your life?	⓪ Not at all noticeable	① A little	② Somewhat	③ Much	④ Very noticeable
⑥ How **worried/distressed** are you about your current sleep problem?	⓪ Not at all worried	① A little	② Somewhat	③ Much	④ Very worried
⑦ To what extent do you consider your sleep problem to **interfere** with your daily functioning (e.g., daytime fatigue, mood, ability to function at work/chores, concentration)?	⓪ Not at all interfering	① A little	② Somewhat	③ Much	④ Very much interferring

Scoring and interpretation

Add the scores for all seven items:
Questions 1 + 2 + 3 + 4 + 5 + 6 + 7 = your total score

Total score categories:

0 to 7	No clinically significant insomnia
8 to 14	Subthreshold insomnia
15 to 21	Clinical insomnia (moderate severity)
22 to 28	Clinical insomnia (severe)

The Insomnia Severity Index (ISI) has seven questions, and you score each one. Then you add the seven scores to get your total score. Compare your score with the guide on page 63.

Prevalence

The most prevalent sleep disorder, insomnia, affects one of every three people in the United States. The Sleep Health Foundation of Australia reported an estimated prevalence rate of 34.5 percent of adults. A TNS Health Care European panel conducted an extensive study in six European countries—the United Kingdom, Spain, the Netherlands, France, Germany, and Italy. Of the approximately 240,000 who completed a self-report survey, 14 percent in the Netherlands and Italy; 20 percent in the United Kingdom, Germany, and Spain; and 26 percent in France reported insomnia symptoms.

Insomnia in younger adults typically manifests as difficulty going to sleep, whereas in older adults insomnia manifests as difficulty staying sleep. If you have ever experienced divorce, lost a job, or lost a family member, chances are that you had trouble going to sleep or staying asleep, which are two of five insomnia patterns. These five insomnia patterns are as follows:

① Inability to fall asleep

② Inability to stay asleep

③ Waking early in the morning

④ Not feeling renewed or refreshed after sleeping

⑤ Feeling as though your sleep is of poor quality or is nonrestorative

These sleep patterns affect your ability to function each day. Most likely, you wake up tired and this makes you less mentally alert. However, most insomniacs do not feel sleepy (as in drowsy or tired). They will complain of fatigue, as if they have no energy and have to push themselves to get things done.

A quick onset of insomnia is called acute adjustment insomnia. Fifteen percent of those with bouts of acute adjustment insomnia (see below) eventually go on to suffer from chronic insomnia. In addition to adjustment insomnia, insomnia of short term or brief duration is also known as acute insomnia, stress-related insomnia, or transient insomnia, and symptoms appear for less than three months, cause considerable concern, and are linked to an identifiable stressor. The primary factor in the diagnosis of insomnia of short duration is whether the sleep disorder becomes an independent focus for the patient. Short-term insomnia typically resolves when the stressor resolves or when the individual adapts to the stressor.

Acute Adjustment Insomnia

Christopher was a forty-one-year-old male and a visiting professor at a university. He had recently lost his brother in an auto accident. Christopher and his brother Leland were only two years apart in age. Although each of them was married and had children of his own, they remained close. Christopher came to the sleep center, and I understood he was experiencing a sleep disorder called acute adjustment insomnia when he explained his predicament.

He wasn't sleeping much. His brother had died tragically and he was in mourning. He took a new position at the university for a change of scenery. When he went to sleep, he saw Leland in a wrecked car or in his casket or saw his dead body on the highway. Christopher tried to distract himself with other tasks and talked with his wife about his grief. He visited my office after seeing an article I wrote on sleep and grief.

Christopher was living through a phase of transient or acute adjustment insomnia. His grief had become all-consuming and even intrusive at night. I was glad Christopher came to the sleep clinic before his insomnia became chronic.

I gave Christopher an initial two-week prescription for a sleep aid to use only if he was unable to fall asleep after several hours. Restorative sleep could improve the physical and mental stressors that Christopher was experiencing.

Early intervention is incredibly important for patients such as Christopher, but a short-term medication is only step one of a larger coping process. If Christopher had continued to go without sleep and still worried and ruminated, the acute condition could have developed into chronic insomnia associated with depression. If he did not address his insomnia, he could see a higher likelihood of developing post-traumatic stress disorder. My goal was to help Christopher start again with sleep habits and rituals that supported his health. We began with sleep hygiene, stimulus control, and a cognitive behavioral therapy for insomnia (CBTI) technique called cognitive restructuring.

Characteristics of Cognitive Intrusions

Intrusive thoughts are distinct, recurring, unwanted, and negative thoughts. The basis of intrusive thoughts in insomnia stems from dysfunctional beliefs about sleep. Intrusive thoughts frequently give birth to worry. People often perceive worry as a way to avoid danger, but at the same time, worry is uncontrollable. You don't plan for intrusive thoughts. They interfere with what you do and how you feel. Cognitive intrusions result in negative moods, and they frequently are a main cause of chronic insomnia. Such intrusions arise for anyone who has a predisposition to ruminate or worry, is overly emotional or sensitive, and has a high intolerance to distress. We become victims of our negative, dysfunctional thoughts.

When stress becomes chronic, you are more susceptible to cognitive intrusions because of the effect stress has on your basic brain chemistry. Your receptors to dopamine, serotonin, norepinephrine, and melatonin become less responsive as stressors increase. This, in turn, renders you psychologically susceptible to intrusive thoughts and insomnia. Also, the connection between your orbitofrontal cortex and your emotional brain center, the amygdala, weakens. Thus, your amygdala is hyperactive and unencumbered by rational thinking.

For example, a college instructor named Linda shared with me that she now recognizes that she does not sleep well despite her initial perceptions that she has slept well. When Linda was a doctoral student, she stayed up late often and eventually experienced insomnia. At that time, she experienced negative cognitive intrusions. The content focused on keeping on top of doctoral work and maintaining a happy marriage. Such was her chronic stress.

Working with a sleep specialist, Linda learned about her dysfunctional beliefs about sleep.

> ## When stress becomes chronic, you are more susceptible to cognitive intrusions because of the effect stress has on your basic brain chemistry.

Throughout the day, she would blame her poor sleep for any problems she had. The sleep specialist had her challenge these negative thoughts with more realistic thoughts and positive affirmations. Also, the sleep specialist helped Linda retrain her sleep habits. She established a consistent sleep schedule, allowing time to relax before going to bed, and wrote out her thoughts in a daily diary. Refocusing her attention to relaxation and winding down from her day had significant effects.

Five years later, Linda, then a college professor, recognized cognitive intrusions were happening again. The content involved negative thoughts about her husband, Dave. Such thoughts were not acceptable to her because they appeared out of nowhere and for no reason that she could identify. She initially ignored the thoughts until their intensity grew and occurred one day while she was in her kitchen chopping vegetables. As the angry thoughts about her husband amplified, Linda's chopping became more intense. Then she noted that the same negative thoughts, which she had control over, reappeared as she was attempting to fall asleep.

Linda understood that her perceptions of the thoughts determined her emotional responses. To change her thoughts to more realistic, balanced thinking would relieve these intrusions. To understand Linda's cognitive intrusions and reframe them, it was important to do the following:

- Appraise the content.
- Define the triggers.
- Determine her ability to control the process.

In appraising the content, Linda discovered that it reflected her feeling overloaded at work and overwhelmed with home chores and daily upkeep. Since she and her husband are the only two people in the home, her husband was the natural target of the content. Her triggers were being tired after a long day and having to make dinner, as well as other chores that needed immediate attention. Linda learned that she could control the process by refocusing her mind on her activities at the moment, rather than worrying about what else needed to be done, and shifting her mood by listening to upbeat music when she worked at home. She learned that trying to distract herself made her feel better, but did not stop the thoughts. She also used a practical, rational approach to self-talk if she felt challenged by the intrusive thoughts. Scrutinizing each thought worked better as a proactive solution. Linda's rational approach included these steps:

1. If Linda had not slept well the previous night,

she paid more attention to what she was thinking during periods of activity such as showering, listing goals for the day, cooking, driving, and reading. She also noted how irritated or angry she felt if she allowed intrusive thoughts to continue without her intervention.

(2) Next she wrote out the thoughts so she could confront them and use a rational approach to counter the effects. Here is one example:

Intrusive thought: *"I am the only one who works hard around here."*

Scrutinize: What does "working hard mean?" To Linda, it reflected the time spent in household activities. She was the chief cook and the one who cleaned up the kitchen every day. This could take between three and five hours per day; on the other hand, her husband ate and left.

Rational Approach: Is this an accurate statement? Linda made the following rational observations:

- *I could spend less time with the kitchen duties if I choose to.*
- *I told Joseph a long time ago how I loved to cook and bragged about how I could manage this part of our relationship.*
- *I am resentful because my time for all the duties I've acquired is short.*
- *I don't manage time as well as I want to. I want help, but I have not asked for help. Realistically, I could afford to hire help.*

(3) What followed Linda's scrutiny and writing were sharing her negative thoughts and realizations with her husband. They commu-nicated well together. Linda was able to ask for help, and their mutual decision was to hire a helper for house cleaning, errands, and cooking two days a week. This helped both of them to spend more time together as well.

Your Thoughts about Sleep Affect Your Sleep
Simply knowing or thinking that you aren't sleeping enough may be a primary reason you can't seem to get adequate sleep. A study published in the *Journal of Experimental Psychology* tested the effects of being told you're getting enough sleep. First, participating Colorado College undergraduates reported how deeply they'd slept the night before, on a scale of 1 to 10. Next, researchers offered a five-minute lesson about sleep's effect on cognitive function. During the lesson, they said that adults normally spend between 20 and 25 percent of their sleep time in REM sleep, getting less than 25 percent REM sleep tends to cause lower performance on learning tests, and getting more than 25 percent REM sleep tends to cause higher performance on tests.

Participants were told that their pulse, heart rate, and brainwave frequency would be measured; in truth, only brainwave frequency was measured. They were told that these measurements would allow the researchers to determine how much REM sleep they'd gotten the night before. This was not true.

Participants were told they got either 16 percent REM sleep or 29 percent REM sleep the previous evening. Then they took a test that measures "auditory attention and speed of processing, skills most affected by sleep deprivation." A second experiment repeated these conditions, while controlling for experiment bias.

Participants who were told they had above-average REM sleep performed better on the test, and those who were told their REM sleep was below average performed worse, even when researchers controlled for the subjects' self-reported sleep quality. If your mindset is that you're well-rested, your brain will perform better, regardless of the actual quality of your sleep. Conversely, constantly talking about how tired you are might be detrimental to your performance.

Treatments for Insomnia

No one solution is right for all patients struggling with insomnia. A sleep doctor can evaluate your needs to determine the best treatment plan for you. Medication options include over-the-counter sleep aids or drugs that regulate the release of neurotransmitters. The medications target the areas of the brain that promote relaxation and reduce anxiety. Newer agents, such as Suvorexant, inhibit the ability of wake-promoting neurotransmitters to act on their target receptor sites. Behavioral solutions such as cognitive behavioral therapies focus on managing stress and anxiety in positive ways. The goals include promoting good sleep hygiene and facilitating restful sleep. Relaxation techniques, breathing techniques, and cognitive behavioral therapies help eliminate sleep-preventing behaviors and thoughts. The new frontier of insomnia treatment is nutritional therapy.

Establishing Proper Sleep Hygiene

Establishing good sleep habits, also called sleep hygiene, refers to the rituals or practices that help you go to sleep and stay asleep. Christopher, in our example above, made several adjustments to his sleep hygiene to ensure better quality sleep.

First, he set a regular sleep schedule. Christopher went to bed at 10 p.m. and woke by 7 a.m. The goal was to reset his body's natural clock and foster better sleep lasting seven to nine hours.

Regular daily exercise helped Christopher diffuse the effects of worry and stressors. To help you plan an exercise program like Christopher's, consider the following: thirty minutes daily of moderate aerobic exercise could include combinations of running, biking, swimming, jumping rope, walking on a treadmill, or using an elliptical machine. Moderate exercise means you can carry on a conversation while exercising. Exercise in the early morning is best for promoting sleep, but evening exercise is better at promoting sleep than no exercise at all. The old bugaboo about evening exercise and elevated body temperature has been shown to be more myth than truth in the latest studies. (See chapter 13 for more on exercise.)

Christopher made the bedroom a restful area. He removed the television and a small computer desk from the bedroom. He added a layer of pull-down shades to the drapes, which were closed at night. The room was considerably darker, and that helped Christopher sleep better. He also kept the bedroom temperature at 68°F (20°C).

Christopher alternated between two relaxation rituals to use before going to sleep. He enjoyed relaxation exercises. On alternative evenings, he lis-

Example of Cognitive Restructuring

Dysfunctional thought	Mood	Transformed by evidential thinking
My brother must have suffered a lot in that accident.	Sad, teary	This isn't true. He died instantly. The officer at the scene said he did not suffer.
I wonder what my brother's final thoughts were.	Scared	The images I see when I go to bed are only projections of my grief. I can transform thoughts of a suffering brother into one who is happy in the afterlife.
I never got to say goodbye, and I never will.	Profoundly sad, heartbroken	I can say goodbye to him now. I can tell him that I miss him and love him.

tened to relaxing music or a meditation exercise. Besides relaxation, Christopher discovered that the meditation exercise helped him cope better with images of his brother that popped up now and then.

Our aim was to reverse the hyperarousal that Christopher developed in response to his bedroom. When Christopher got into bed, his mind raced, he felt anxious, and he was unable to fall asleep. He had taken to lying in bed and trying to make himself fall asleep, which would not work and led to more frustration.

Stimulus Control Therapy

Stimulus control therapy is an effective method for managing insomnia and must be used consistently. Christopher was instructed to go to bed only when he felt sleepy. He went to bed at 10 p.m. each night, but could not always fall asleep within twenty minutes in the beginning of his new routine. When he couldn't, he got out bed and went to the den to read until he felt sleepy, which was his signal to return to bed. He repeated this process as necessary.

Sometimes Christopher wanted to nap in the afternoon and this would decrease his drive to fall asleep at night. I instructed Christopher in how napping, especially for more than an hour, reduces the pressure that builds up during the day to fall asleep. In sleep medicine, we call this buildup during the day the homeostatic drive to sleep. So he did not nap, as part of controlling his schedule and retraining his habits. If he absolutely had to nap, he was instructed to limit naps to twenty minutes.

Cognitive Restructuring

Cognitive restructuring in an acute case such as Christopher's is about identifying and challenging the spontaneous thoughts that occur when you

Example of stressor thought and feeling	Reframe positively as acceptance and fact
Thought: It is already midnight and I'll never get to sleep now.	**Fact (a simple statement):** I'm not sleepy right now. That's okay. I won't worry about it.
Emotion: The whole neighborhood is sleeping but I am not. I hate this.	**Consequence (a statement of action):** I am going to get up and continue reading until I am sleepy again.

are distressed or sleep deprived. In more chronic cases of insomnia, it is also about recognizing and changing the dysfunctional maladaptive beliefs about sleep that you have developed. The challenge and subsequent rational evidence to dispute unhealthy thinking enabled Christopher's breakthrough in reducing intense anxiety levels. For example, consider how stressed Christopher was at his brother's funeral and during the following weeks. He explained he felt numb. When he thought he could sleep and relax, he couldn't. Rather, he started thinking about how his brother died. Then different thoughts sneaked in: His brother was scared. His brother suffered. Christopher would be lonely. His stress response had evolved into a state of chronic alert or hyperarousal, and such negative thoughts would worsen if he did not change them.

Christopher followed this advice to help change his thought patterns:

⟫ Be calm during this process. Try to relax.
⟫ Focus on one topic (for Christopher, one aspect of his brother's death).
⟫ Write down any thoughts that arise.

⟫ For each automatic thought, write the mood it triggered.
⟫ When finished writing those thoughts, refute each thought by writing the contradiction. This helps balance any irrational thinking.
⟫ Read each contradiction aloud to hear as well as see each statement, and then record how moods shifted, if they did.
⟫ Practice this exercise for twenty minutes daily in the evening for two weeks.

Christopher reported that during the first week of the writing exercises he mentally argued with himself about how this "silly exercise" wouldn't bring Leland back. During the second week he practiced cognitive restructuring, he could laugh at his racing thoughts, urging him to ditch the "useless exercise." He got the point. He laughed again. This is when he knew he would survive and accept how Leland died.

Continuing this practice helps de-escalate the hyperarousal by reframing faulty thinking associated with going to bed. This practice also produces calmer emotions and allows for better sleep habits. The benefit of this approach is that you will have more energy, as opposed to distress and anxiety depleting your energy. You are being proactive! You gain insight into what your dysfunctional thoughts are and how you can change your thoughts and change your moods.

Cognitive Behavioral Therapy for Insomnia

In sleep medicine, I prefer the use of cognitive behavioral therapy for insomnia (CBTI) to medications when possible. CBTI is a form of psychotherapy or counseling, with varied techniques to help you regulate thoughts as well as behaviors. CBTI is used for persistent insomnia as the primary disorder, as well as with coexisting disorders.

Insomnia is the more prevalent of sleep disorders and associated with high-stress lifestyles or anxiety behaviors. Consequently, I see many patients who have been on sleep medications for years. Their prescriptions no longer work. Some patients express a strong desire to avoid taking medications or want to discontinue them for reasons such as daytime sleepiness or fear of getting dependent on them. They wish to know about alternative choices to drugs. The goals for better sleep are as follows:

⟩ To reverse behaviors that prevent sleep

⟩ To restructure or retrain thinking and attitudes about sleep

⟩ To maintain a consistent sleep/wake schedule with the emphasis on a set wake time

In CBTI, we work on negative thinking patterns such as worry or rumination. On page 69 to 70 you read about replacing negative thoughts with positive, realistic ones, such as:

⟩ "I've been through this before, and I'm able to function."

⟩ "I know that most people with insomnia tend to underestimate the amount of sleep they actually get."

⟩ "I can control unhealthy thinking by writing down my worries and emptying my mind."

Although the goal with CBTI is to see a change in behavior, it is not enough to change only the behavior. The ability to solidify new habits means changing the way you think about yourself and what you experience in life. For example, you may learn how to assert yourself on the job (behavior), but do you inherently believe that you will succeed? You must change how you think (cognition) about your abilities to accomplish the goal. In other words, you must feel confident and believe you are competent in the situation to sustain transformation.

Unfortunately, brains have a tendency toward cognitive bias, or the propensity to look at situations negatively rather than positively. Therefore, only bad things seem to happen to you. You draw the wrong conclusions or make illogical choices, perpetuating the cycle. To break this pattern, it is vital that you make a commitment to achieve your best sleep and health.

In CBTI, the focus is on learning to stop automatic negative thinking/thoughts. Next, you learn to replace them with positive thoughts that become habitual. As we read on page 69, there is a direct correlation between what you think and how your body feels. To modify your sleep habits, set up good habits and avoid bad habits. See chapter 4 for helpful strategies.

If you go to bed expecting to sleep and don't

go to sleep right away, how does your mind react? How does your body feel? Tackling the psychological focus on going to sleep challenges your cognitive biases about sleep. The CBTI approach is to break the link between your thoughts and how you feel. Otherwise, your thoughts about the lack of sleep negatively affect your ability to sleep and can increase stress and anxiety. Some insomniacs develop numerous dysfunctional beliefs about sleep, such as these:

⟫ "I know if I don't sleep for nine hours, I'll be miserable all week."
⟫ "Insomnia makes me not think clearly at work and do dumb things."
⟫ "I just know I won't be able to function."
⟫ "I'm going to lose my job."

These negative thoughts and counterproductive behaviors stimulate more stress hormones, making sleepless nights even worse. A sleep specialist may challenge the dysfunctional beliefs in friendly ways: "Let's get a reality check. Show me the evidence for that belief. Let's track your sleep patterns in a sleep diary and see if that thought plays out." The point is to get you to observe your thoughts, record them, and change them. Then you are accountable to report progress and the findings with the sleep expert.

This cognitive restructuring challenges you to validate the reality by introducing a fact and consequence. The purpose is to take the pressure off and redirect your self-blame into a positive scenario. Acceptance, rather than frustration, is a better mechanism to reduce stressful thinking and encourage relaxation exercises or sleep restriction therapy.

CBTI changes incorrect or habitual thoughts that lead to emotional suffering. A diary or record of the thoughts and feelings helps you identify and change the habits that do not work for you.

Medications

The U.S. Federal Drug Administration has approved several classes of medications for the treatment of insomnia. Although I do not believe this is necessarily the best approach, it is important to understand how these drugs work.

⟫ **Over-the-counter sleep aids** are typically antihistamines that block histamine, a stimulating, wake-promoting neurotransmitter. Undesirable side effects include constipation, urinary retention, dry mouth, daytime sedation, and increased risk of Alzheimer's. They lose effectiveness after a short time, as users become more tolerant of the drug.

> *Acceptance, rather than frustration, is a better mechanism to reduce stressful thinking and encourage relaxation exercises or sleep restriction therapy.*

> **Melatonin supplements** shorten the time to fall asleep and are effective in certain circadian disorders, such as jet lag or delayed sleep onset. Also, melatonin can be effective for the elderly who tend to produce less of it. Beta blockers such as propranolol and metoprolol are commonly prescribed for hypertension, heart disease, tremors, and migraines. However, because they can also block the production of melatonin by the pineal gland, they can cause insomnia. As a result, we are now seeing more physicians prescribing melatonin when patients on these medications develop problems with falling and staying asleep.

> **Benzodiazepines** are medications that target gamma-aminobutyric acid (GABA), the most potent sleep-promoting neurotransmitter in the brain. Benzodiazepines, including temazepam, triazolam, flurazepam, and diazepam, make this GABA neurotransmitter more efficient. They also work on anxiety, memory, muscle-relaxing, and seizure-inhibiting receptors. This is likely why withdrawal is more prevalent. Do note that a recent study of people on benzodiazepines demonstrated an increased likelihood of developing Alzheimer's in those over age sixty. Those who were on the benzodiazepines for longer than 180 days increased the risk of Alzheimer's by 84 percent.

> **Non-benzodiazepines**, including zolpidem and eszopiclone, also target the GABA system, but they have a different chemical structure and interact predominantly with receptors for sleep. They promote sleep better than older, nonselective benzodiazepines. However, zolpidem has been found to intensify negative emotional memories. A recent study in Taiwan indicated an increased incidence of non-Alzheimer's dementia in older individuals who took between 170 and 800 mg of zolpidem per year.

> **Medications not developed for sleep**, yet commonly used for sleep, though the FDA has not approved them, include antidepressants such as trazodone, amitriptyline, and mirtazapine and the antipsychotic medication quetiapine.

My recommendation is to begin with CBTI to achieve better sleep. However, some patients with severe physiological hyperarousal may require medication. In those cases, I try to avoid benzodiazepines. I will occasionally use non-benzodiazepines. However, trazodone and low-dose doxepin are preferable. Ramelton is a medication unlike any of the others because it works on the melatonin receptors in the hypo-thalamus. Ramelteon is the safest medication and associated with the fewest side effects. In addition, a 2003 study found that doxepin lowered the cortisol levels of insomniacs. Seek the advice of your physician before taking sleep medication or deciding on which medication is best for you.

Cannabis for Sleep and Anxiety

When it comes to sleep and anxiety, alleviating symptoms through the use of marijuana has been poorly studied and is confusing at best. Much of the information available is anecdotal. However, we know that the human brain and body is full of receptor sites called cannabinoid receptors. Our bodies produce endocannabinoids, which work on these receptors, and when we smoke marijuana or take synthetic medications derived from constitu-ents of marijuana, it also works on these receptors.

The clinical effects of smoking marijuana are frequently muddled by the psychotropic high that results. A few studies tout marijuana sativa, or indica, or hybrids of the two for sleep-related issues. However, they are poorly done and anecdotal.

On the other hand, studies performed using synthetically derived components of the marijuana plant such as nabilone (Cesamet) and cannabidiol are rather impressive. These studies have shown significant responses to nabilone in patients with PTSD-related insomnia as well as nightmares. Other studies have shown

improvement in anxiety with cannabidiol.

At this point, it would appear that the synthetic derivatives, which selectively activate cannabi-noid receptors, hold the greatest promise in the treatment of insomnia, nightmares, and anxiety. Marijuana in the commonly smoked form would appear to work for some people. However, when discontinued, a severe rebound in the form of insomnia and nightmares may occur. The FDA, for example, would not release a sleeping pill that commonly resulted in severe rebound insomnia. So I believe the future lies in further studies of synthetic derivatives.

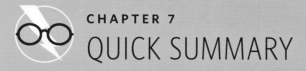

CHAPTER 7
QUICK SUMMARY

》 Insomnia refers to the inability to go to sleep, stay asleep, or waking earlier than normal in the morning.

》 Those with insomnia share traitssuch as hyperarousal, difficulty in coping, worrying, or ruminating.

》 Intrusive negative thoughts and dysfunctional beliefs about sleep are two symptoms of those experiencing insomnia.

》 Managing these behaviors through cognitive behavioral therapy for insomnia is effective.

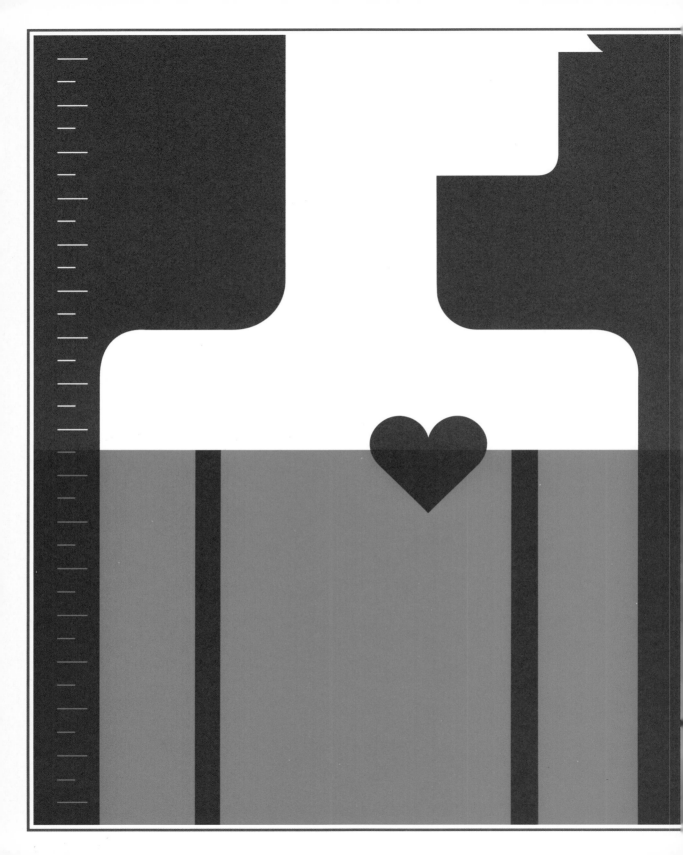

CHAPTER 8

UNDERSTANDING AND REDUCING STRESS AND ANXIETY

The basic chemistry of stressors, the activation of the hypothalamus-pituitary-adrenal (HPA) axis, is the same mechanism that drives distress, anxiety, and panic. You can manage stressors if you are alert to psychological changes and physical symptoms or behaviors when you get stressed. Recognize when you have crossed over from stress to trying repeatedly to manage stressors so you can avoid transitioning to distress. This section explains the escalations or transitions and how you can identify feelings or behaviors characterizing stress, distress, anxiety, and panic.

Don't let stress hijack your health or your enthusiasm for living. You've read how the fight-or-flight pattern, the hyperarousal of the nervous system, is our basic survival instinct, but you do not want to live in that state for twenty-four hours of the day. The problem is that prolonged, heightened states of stress take their toll on sleep, health, cognitive function, and immune system health, to name a few. You have to know what you are dealing with to eliminate the cause or to be more proactive in managing stress. You can approach stress in a variety of productive ways:

- ❱ Change your unhealthy thinking and how you believe stress affects you.
- ❱ Choose new ways to manage your lifestyle effectively.
- ❱ Get rid of the cause of the stress.

Develop Your Personal Stress Profile

One method to determine which types of stress you experience and how you respond to stress and self-care is to develop a personal stress profile. The assessments, charts, and checklists throughout this book will provide you the feedback you need. Complete the following charts to create your stress profile.

Indicators of stress levels are a faster pulse and higher breathing rate. Chest breathing, or thoracic breathing, means your breaths are shallow. Deeper breathing involves the diaphragm and abdominal muscles, and it relaxes you.

To confirm a definite stressor pattern, you can measure the physical manifestations of stress that you experience in two ways. The first chart is a list of symptoms, and you fill in the frequency of the symptoms based on what you remember.

The second approach is to keep a reaction

Personal Stress Profile: Physical Symptoms—Normal vs. Sample Response (Female, age 60, may have insomnia)

Physiology	Assessment	Normal	Sample response
Breathing pattern	Do you breathe from your ○ Chest ○ Abdomen ○ Both	Chest breathing is a sign of stress. Diaphragmatic or abdominal breathing is relaxing.	Chest
Breathing rate	_____ breaths per minute	12 to 16	21
Resting heart rate	_____ beats per minute	Average adult rate is 70 to 80 beats per minute.	80

Personal Stress Profile Summary

Now fill out the assessment above for yourself. The chart below identifies stress indicators.

	Chest or abdominal breather	Breaths per minute	Resting heart rate
Write your score			
Stress indicators (mark one)	○ Chest (high stress) ○ Abdominal (normal)	○ High (over 16) ○ Normal ○ Low (under 12)	○ High (over 80) ○ Normal ○ Low (under 70)

diary for two to four weeks. This period is long enough for you to recognize your stress reaction patterns. If you commit to keeping a log of physical stress symptoms, seeing the daily log makes it hard for you to deny the symptoms. The technique works wonders when my patients can see the patterns and take back control to achieve better sleep results.

You now have two types of stress scores: events that cause you stress and how often you react to those stressors. You have also identified sleep issues that affect stress and stressors that affect sleep. This information is your stress profile.

How to Prioritize and Plan Your Stress Management Solutions

Now that you've completed your stress profile, it's time to choose ideas and activities for a more relaxed lifestyle and better sleep. None of these activities is a quick fix. Yet, the step-by-step

Frequency and Consistency of Physical Stress Manifestations

	Seems like all day, every day	Once or twice daily	Every night and day	Two to four times per week	Once per week	Several times per month	Never
Feeling irritable or grouchy							
Headaches							
Tense muscles in shoulders, neck, or back							
Fatigue, exhaustion, or listlessness							
Gut discomfort							
Eating less or minimally, not very hungry							
Overeating							
Cramps, gas, constipation							
Taking one hour or more to fall to sleep							
Waking up earlier than normal consistently							
Bouts of anger or hostility							
Feeling boredom, sadness, or gloominess							
Worry or anxiety							

Daily Log of Stress Events

	Mon.	Tues.	Wed.	Thurs.	Fri.	Sat.	Sun.
Physical symptoms							
Breathing faster							
Tense muscles							
Headache							
Difficulty focusing							
Restless							
Bowel problems							
Emotional symptoms							
Irritable							
Anxious							
Angry							
Impatient							
Hopeless							
Behavior							
Can't relax or settle in							
Insomnia and sleep disturbances							
Arguing, nitpicking							
Busy but not productive							
Crying							
Increase in alcohol use, smoking, or drug use							

Fill in the frequency or number of occurrences for each symptom every evening. At the end of the week, determine whether you are accurate in identifying your stress responses and how often they occur.

approach will help you focus on the topic and then take action to reduce distress and anxiety. Here are the three steps:

1. Tackle the problem.

2. Take care of your mind.

3. Take care of your body.

Step 1: Tackle the Problem

Most people ignore problems and push them away. But when problems are "out of sight and out of mind," it does not mean they are gone. In fact, because you know the problems are there, you worry more and stay awake more. I enjoy using the word *tackle* to approach a problem. The word reminds patients of a husky, well-padded football giant, who brings the player carrying the football to the ground. Envision that you can tackle the source of stress successfully. Bring it to the ground! This exercise gives you emotional strength to fix the problem and gain confidence in taking action.

Start by listing the top five stressors in your life right now (see worksheet in Appendix C, page 147). Are those stressors about people, work you have to do, topics you worry about, or a situation that causes emotional reactions? After you've listed the problems, brainstorm ideas for tackling them.

Tackle the work or tasks first. Ask for help if you need support. Put the task on your calendar daily and remind yourself by posting sticky notes where you will see them or use your phone or computer's reminder system. You are training your brain and body to accept the chore and not increase stress. Get it done!

If the work or task overwhelms you, remember that writing down the steps to completion will get the worries out of your mind and onto paper. Break a large task down into smaller, progressive steps and number them in the order to complete. Just do step one today to make the work less overwhelming. This helps you sleep better, too, because you won't worry about whether you can do it all. You have tackled the first task, and you'll realize that you can handle the next and then the next.

Step 2: Take Care of Your Mind

The next three practices help patients diffuse stress and sleep better.

Avoid stressors when possible. Consider how to identify and avoid stressors to diffuse your reactions or to prevent incidents that trigger your stress. Knowing how to manage stressors involves two essential points: taming your reactivity to stress and making tough choices to avoid stressful situations when possible.

Start journaling to ease stress. See suggestions below for stress-related journal topics. Write about one of the topics that worries you, and then tear up the paper and throw it away.

- Which people will you talk with about boundaries?
- Do you need to cancel or reschedule any activities?
- What do you worry about that you cannot change?

Use positive self-talk. Say to yourself, "There is nothing I can do to change circumstances I can't control. I will no longer drain my energy by worrying about them. I will fix the circumstances I can. I will not take on anyone else's stress."

Step 3: Take Care of Your Body

Make exercise your top priority. The stress response mobilizes you to move, fight, or run. Take the opportunity to release tension through movement. How do you enjoy movement? Take a short run or a brisk power walk. Walk the dog and relax outdoors. Dance and exercise to salsa or merengue.

If you are distressed about an upcoming test or work assignment, don't dive in and push yourself harder. First, relax or exercise to clear your mind. Pushing harder causes more distress and makes it harder to think clearly. Exercise first to diffuse pent-up energy so you can focus better.

When you are overwhelmed with work or tasks, do you push through or take breaks? Do you work through lunch? To break stressful patterns, you have to do the opposite of your inclination. Instead of hunching at your desk or straining your eyes to gaze at a bright computer screen, get up, stretch, and drink water to stay hydrated. Researchers have found that taking a walk outdoors or using a treadmill benefits your brain. Exercise increases threefold an essential protein called brain-derived neurotrophic factor (BDNF) that is crucial for growing and maintaining healthy neurons, or brain cells. Imagine how the exercise and resulting healthy cells could stave off neurological problems and disease. Another major benefit is reduced stress. (See chapter 13 for more on exercise.)

Also, make sure you eat breakfast every morning and include a source of protein, which helps keep your blood sugar balanced and provides energy for your day. To manage your stress effectively, you need to eat nutritious foods.

Eliminate refined carbohydrates (sugary foods and drinks) from your diet and replace them with meals containing whole grains. Refined carbohydrates either lack or have been stripped of fiber. This results in a rapid elevation of blood sugar that elicits a stress response with the overproduction of insulin followed by a cortisol dump. This is the body's attempt to bring your sugar back up from the low induced by too much insulin. This process begins a detrimental cycle that continues all day and night if you eat a diet of simple carbohydrates.

You may know already that good nutrition keeps your moods balanced and eating regularly keeps your mind alert. Below is a list of foods that decrease distress and produce a calming effect. This effect is not the sleepy, foggy carbohydrate effect that results from comfort foods.

Calming foods provide energy or have nutrients that soothe an overworked system. Because of the specific nutrients they provide and the steady, reliable source of energy they give you, they'll get you through the day feeling focused and balanced:

⟆ Asparagus has large amounts of folic acid that stabilizes moods.

⟆ Avocados have beta-carotene, vitamin E, and more folic acid. Beta-carotene and vitamin E are antioxidants that protect cell membranes and nerve cells from oxidative stress.

⟆ Berries such as strawberries, blueberries, raspberries, and blackberries, are rich in vitamin C, which is helpful in decreasing excessive cortisol production.

⟆ Nuts, especially cashews, are a smart protein source for snacking. Cashews contain zinc,

> "True good health is a state of dynamic well-being, one that is like that of childhood exuberance and joy, boundless energy, keen awareness of surroundings, positive emotional state and a natural love and zest for life."
>
> —William Wolcott and Trish Fahey, authors of popular nutrition books

which is helpful for people with anxiety or depression, both of which correlate to low zinc levels. Almonds are also helpful for ingesting more vitamin B₂, vitamin E, magnesium, and zinc.

⟫ Whole-grain foods can have a powerful calming effect on anxiety and contain beneficial nutrients. Look for grains such as whole wheat, brown rice, amaranth, and quinoa. Whole-grain cereals include steel-cut oats, rolled oats, barley, and buckwheat. They are excellent sources of B vitamins and magnesium.

For more on food and anxiety, see chapter 9.

Sleeping Better

This part of your stress resolution plan is making a commitment to developing better sleep habits. Consider the following plan to sleep well each night:

⟫ You need seven to nine hours of sleep each night. Determine what time you should be in bed and ready for sleep by setting a wake time. This is the time you'll get out of bed every morning.

⟫ Avoid caffeine six to eight hours before going to bed.

⟫ Finish chores or other tasks at least one hour before bed.

⟫ Take a hot shower or warm bath to help you relax.

⟫ Find a quiet place in your home to sit or relax in some way and release the emotional tension. If you are troubled or upset more than usual, then increase your time to wind down.

⟫ Dim the lights about sixty minutes before going to bed.

Improve Self-Esteem to Combat Stress

Healthy self-esteem is based on your ability to assess yourself accurately and accept and value yourself without conditions or reservations. How you see yourself becomes a self-fulfilling prophecy. For example, if you feel undeserving, the likelihood of attaining your desire or ending up in a relationship that you value is diminished.

Transform negative beliefs into positive

ones by writing about your experiences. There are several ways you can accomplish this:

- ⟩ Start by making a list of tasks you do well now and tasks that you've successfully completed in the past.
- ⟩ Each morning, write down a brief story of several paragraphs on one thing you have done well.
- ⟩ Choose one task for the day. Make a commitment to follow through and complete the task. Write this success in a success journal each evening.

Writing a story can help you develop good feelings and positive memories about what you have done in the past. The same is true if you choose to write about a current event in which you succeed. The action can be separate from your thoughts about it. The action is a fact and represents your strength. You may not feel a difference right away. However, writing down these facts each day for one month challenges your assumptions and negative beliefs. Over time, you will notice that you're feeling more confident and that your self-esteem is slowly improving and, in turn, you will develop healthier responses to stress. The following steps can help.

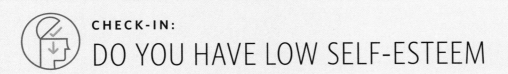

CHECK-IN:
DO YOU HAVE LOW SELF-ESTEEM

○ Do you judge yourself as effective or not effective by the present situation instead of seeing the bigger picture of accomplishments and friendships?

○ Do you blame your failure on others, thinking that what happens to you is because of another person or external circumstances?

○ Do you put yourself down through deprecating words and thoughts?

○ Do you treat yourself badly, or treat yourself worse than you would treat others?

○ Is it hard for you to accept compliments?

○ Do you feel nervous or anxious much of the time?

○ Do you show too much concern for what other people think about you?

○ Do you stress the negatives in situations?

○ Do you neglect activities that you would do for yourself?

○ Do you put yourself last and put others' interests ahead of you?

○ Do you have difficulty finding the value in your strengths and talents?

When you are happy, you encourage others to be happy around you. Happiness is infectious.

Put Yourself First

Put your needs first instead of putting your needs aside to make others happy. There's nothing wrong with wanting to make others happy, and it shows you have a generous heart. But to be happy and improve your self-esteem, your needs must be fulfilled, and you are the only one who can do that. This is not being selfish. Ask yourself: Why should everyone else be happy but you? That doesn't seem fair or sensible.

You deserve to be happy, and you can be happy. Meeting your needs first rather than feeling dissatisfaction and resentment will allow you to be a better person, friend, or family member to others.

☉ **When you are happy, you encourage others to be happy around you. Happiness is infectious.**

Build Your Support System

Find friends who support you in improving your self-esteem. Many of us have friends who fall into different categories: those who find fault in what we do, and those who pick us up when we fall down.

Spending time with people who are critical of your behavior, actions, or appearance is degrading your self-esteem. Avoid these people. Develop friendships that make you feel better, happier, or more positive. Don't forget to write

TERM REVIEW

Stress includes the initial activation of the sympathetic nervous system that increases your heart rate, blood pressure, and breathing. Adrenaline is released to give you an energy edge to challenge or escape the perceived danger.

Distress refers to taxing, painful, insulting, or tiring experiences that drain your energy. Distress interferes with your physiology and can lead to maladaptive behaviors such as withdrawal or aggression. People under constant distress risk higher odds of becoming sick.

Anxiety is excessive and chronic stress reactions to everyday situations. Anxiety can be disabling when it persists and overwhelms you. When anxiety is excessive, you may experience extreme dread or irrational fears of situations that occur every day and seem so normal to others. When such anxiety interferes with your functioning, you've most likely developed an anxiety disorder.

> ## "The key is how often you are feeling this sense of distress, how bad it gets, and how long it lasts; that is what can help determine the seriousness of your situation."
>
> —Abby Aronowitz, Ph.D., the director of SelfHelpDirectives.com

that you took that action as a good, positive step today.

(!) **Remember that you deserve good friends and people who see you in a positive light.**

Escalation from Stress to Distress

When you're unable to properly manage stress, it can escalate to distress or anxiety, even panic. The hyperarousal symptoms start out the same way for stress, distress, and anxiety: Your heart beats faster. You start sweating. Your gut churns a bit. Stress signals that your brain and body need attention.

Distress is a negative emotional reaction when you are not able to manage the stressors. Coping behaviors no longer work. Your body chemistry enters a heightened stressed state, and you're unable to calm down. You have low energy and get little healthful sleep. Getting something done requires that you focus better, work longer, or expend more time or energy to complete a task. You are easily agitated and appear sensitive to your environment.

Distress could signal physical discomfort or pain. Check in with yourself to see if you notice these behaviors: feeling more irritable or tense; noticing more forgetfulness, foggy thinking, or general fatigue; or feeling pressured, out of control, poor at managing time, or bothered by others. Psychological distress is a subjective experience, and an inability to cope or manage it could lead to other symptoms such as unhelpful thinking, increased worry, or rumination.

Solutions may require that you list priorities, solve a problem, ask for help, or take care of your health by seeing a sleep specialist or nutritionist. Two factors, predictability and controllability, can lessen the intensity and duration of your stress symptoms.

When Anxiety Develops

You have, undoubtedly, felt anxious before and experienced symptoms such as excessive worry. Perhaps you felt anxious when you had to ace a big test or prepare for an important interview. These kinds of feelings are normal. Everyone experiences feeling anxious at some point, although the reasons vary—work pressures, finances, loss, and relationship issues, to name a few.

Feeling anxious is normal; it is called anxiety when your distress becomes obsessive worry and apprehension about what could happen or what might happen. The chart below depicts the differences between distress and anxiety behaviors.

Differences between Distress and Anxiety

Anxiety is an internal reaction to the excessive and chronic stress of everyday situations, characterized by worry and apprehension. Even if you use the terms *distress* and *anxiety* interchangeably, it's important to learn to differentiate between the two so you can better manage your symptoms.

Distress escalations and anxiety overload demonstrate hyperarousal of the physical body and brain. You are unable to sleep or relax. Worry and dread interfere with your life. In one sense, this is a point of making wise decisions to support your emotional health and mental health. Visit a sleep specialist, because sleeping is the definite path for healing. You need to learn and manage anxiety when you feel anxious all the time. Otherwise, the anxiety can become so bad that you avoid situations and isolate yourself.

Anxiety and Panic

People often use the words "anxiety attack" and "panic attack" to refer to the same event; however, a panic attack, anxiety attack, and panic disorder are truly different.

Anxiety attack: You might experience an anxiety attack as a result of a stressor, such as the death of a person close to you. You may have a rapid heartbeat and shortness of breath, apprehension, or fear. When the stressor or

Differences between Distress and Anxiety

Distress	Anxiety
The emotional and physical tension that manifests as sleep disturbances, headaches, fatigue, or other physical responses such as neck or muscle tension.	Physical tension escalates to fear, unease, or panic. More autonomic nervous symptoms present as numbness, dry mouth, breathing problems or shortness of breath, and sleep issues.
Related to thoughts or external events that are most stressful when internalized and worrying begins.	Related to internal states of apprehension, expectant danger, and feeling powerless. Nervousness reigns and worries are persistent.
Mental and emotional reactions are like short fuses. You find it hard to control outbursts, even when you are aware of building tension.	Related to internal stress overreactions rather than to an external irritant.
Has roots in frustrations that grow into an inability to manage the emotional overload, and the brain and body start to shut down.	Has roots in fear; when hypervigilance sets in, the focused worry increases. You have trouble concentrating or thinking differently.

cause is gone, then the anxiety attack ends and is usually of short duration. When you have repeated anxiety attacks, the next diagnosis could be an anxiety disorder.

Panic attack: A panic attack's onset is sudden and lasts about ten minutes. People report that they do not incite or provoke a panic attack. If you have a panic attack, you will likely experience intense fear. You may also have pain in your chest, abdomen, or muscles. You feel as if you can't breathe and may also feel sweaty, dizzy, or faint. Many people who have panic attacks feel that they are having a heart attack. The apprehension of another panic attack often alters the individual's lifestyle, leading to a panic disorder.

Panic disorder: Recurrent, unexpected attacks followed by persistent periods in constant fear of another attack characterize a panic disorder. The three psychological symptoms are the feeling of unreality, the fear of dying, and the fear of losing control.

Panic Attacks and Panic Disorder

A panic attack is one form of anxiety disorder. (Anxiety disorders are discussed further in chapter 11.) A hallmark of a panic attack is that it comes on suddenly. For a time, the reason was unclear. Some interesting research has shed light on patients who hyperventilated chronically, which can be a feature of anxiety disorders, and fitted them with twenty-four-hour monitors. One hour before the onset of an attack, the monitors showed physiologic instability. The participants exhibited low carbon dioxide levels, which then rose quickly right before the panic attack and felt like suffocation, anxiety, and fear

of dying. This study explains how the physiologic instabilities create the psychological responses during a panic attack, in addition to the other physical symptoms such as hot flashes, trembling, choking, nausea, and numbness.

Susceptibility to Panic

Health professionals agree that people with a particular temperament are more sensitive to stress or prone to negative emotions. They are more likely to experience anxiety or panic, either of which could develop into a disorder requiring treatment. Now we also know that insomnia and sleep apnea coexist with anxiety and panic. They share the common physiology of hyperarousal and sleep disturbances. Treating the sleep disorder often resolves the psychological issues.

Also, sleep apnea is sometimes misdiagnosed as nocturnal panic attacks. After all, the person with sleep apnea may awaken suddenly feeling short of breath, feeling apprehensive, sweating, and with a rapid heartbeat. However, in the case of sleep apnea, it is a physiological reaction to a closed airway and the resultant struggle to breathe. One clue that it may not be a panic attack and may be sleep apnea is if such episodes always seem to occur during sleep and not during the day.

Those people who are susceptible to panic have the following characteristics:

① Sensitivity to adrenal or hormone changes that include a tendency toward overactive adrenal glands. The overproduction of adrenaline and cortisol interferes with the production of the neurotransmitters that

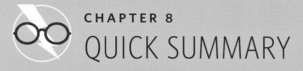

CHAPTER 8

QUICK SUMMARY

> A stress profile involves identifying and learning to manage the stressors in your life. You will understand the basic hyperarousal activation for stress, distress, and anxiety.

> Then you train yourself to recognize signs of escalation, such as intensity, duration, and triggers. The nuggets of knowledge are part of your plan for relief of unhealthy thinking.

> Taking charge again helps you predict and manage lifestyle choices, but first you tackle and solve the stressor, event or problem. Now is your time!

> Because the activation of the hypothalamus-pituitary-adrenal (HPA) axis drives stress reactions and distress, anxiety, and panic, knowing how you react is key to healing. Then choose activities that resonate with you to decrease hyperarousal. Take positive action through exercise. Keeping a journal of your progress helps you mentally clarify your choices and stay optimistic. If you enjoy friendships that support your transformation, ask one good friend to be your accountability partner; this person listens, supports, and provides feedback.

stabilize moods. In fact, persistently high cortisol levels have been found to damage the ability of the receptor sites for serotonin, dopamine, and norepinephrine to respond to their respective neurotransmitters.

② Sensitivity to physical stimuli, such as bright lights, harsh sounds, temperature fluctuations, and extreme temperatures.

③ People prone to panic attacks may have a genetic inclination, with a higher incidence noted in families. Also, a hyperactive amygdala, which overreacts to stimulation from other regions of the brain, may be a major cause. The amygdala stimulates the HPA axis and, in turn, the sympathetic nervous system. Poor sleep tends to intensify this response.

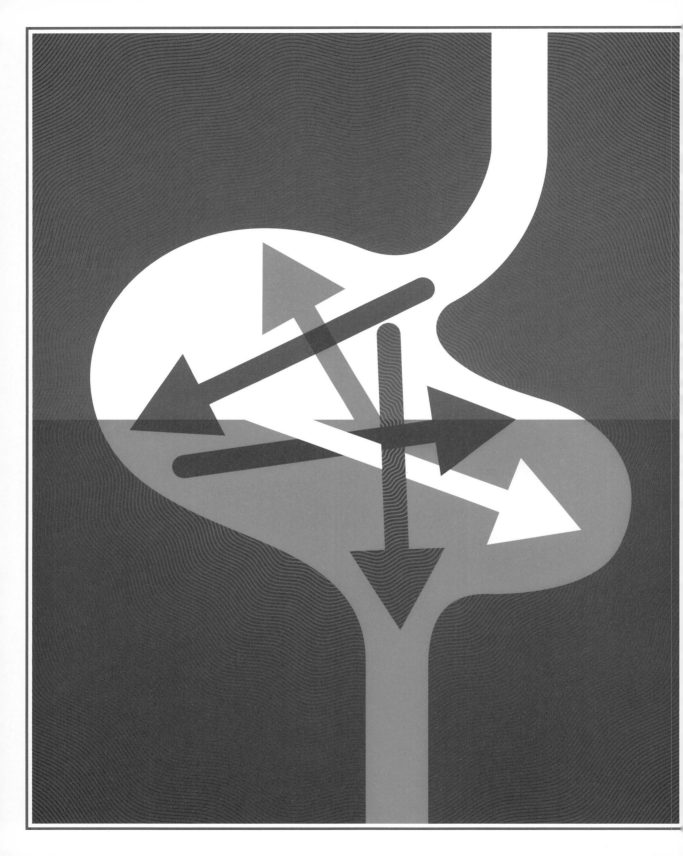

CHAPTER 9

HOW FOOD AFFECTS ANXIETY

When stressors place demands on your brain and body, you lose restraint because of the hyperarousal effect. Many people feel a craving for comfort foods, as they contain the calories of saturated fats and carbohydrates for energy. People with higher cortisol levels in times of stress tend to crave more snack foods, desserts, and sweets. In this context, this type of eating is stress related and driven by cortisol, not an eating disorder.

You are capable of managing emotional eating by making a deliberate decision to avoid sweets and bad carbohydrates that rapidly shoot up your blood sugar. Insightful writing, meditation, or counseling can help you determine and control the triggers.

Characteristics of emotional hunger to watch for include the following:

❭ Cravings that come on fast
❭ Cravings for food that fill an emotional void
❭ Craving instant satisfaction
❭ Eating beyond being full or satisfied

Nutrients

If you are anxious because distress has a grip on you, then focus on the vitamins and minerals that can help keep you calm.

Vitamin C is high in antioxidants. To rebalance the HPA axis and reduce cortisol levels, take vitamin C. Studies show that marathon runners who take 1,500 milligrams a day have significantly lower cortisol levels following their races (stressful event) than those who do not. Runners should take 1,500 milligrams each day for seven days prior to the race, on the day of the race, and two consecutive days after the race.

Likewise, if you have an upcoming event that stresses you, plan ahead and take care of your cortisol. If you have been deprived of sleep and experience impairment of memory, vitamin C repairs the stress. You can find vitamin C in these food sources:

Fruits: Citrus fruits, strawberries, and kiwi

Vegetables: Cabbage, spinach and other leafy greens, tomatoes, potatoes, and green peppers

Omega-3 fatty acids boost mood and help prevent the risk of heart disease. High omega-3 intake also reduces distress symptoms and cortisol secretion.

ARE YOU AN EMOTIONAL EATER?

Eating behavior	Take immediate action	Take control long-term
You respond to cravings at any time without much thought.	When you feel the craving, sip a hot, calming tea.	Keep a diary of emotional triggers when in this stressed phase.
Your cravings are for specific tastes, such as sweet or salty.	Add a natural sweetener to your drink.	When the urge strikes, rate the urge on a scale of 1 (lowest) to 100 (highest). If your rating is over the number 50, say to yourself, "I am here right now and can make a new decision to not overeat/eat poorly. Instead, I will . . . " Then do it!
The craving is repeated.	Add a protein source to the carb for a more balanced snack.	Eat more slowly and chew the protein well. Savor the flavor.
Slow down your eating pattern.	Cut a large portion into much smaller portions, thus requiring a longer time to relax and eat more slowly.	Do your research and find a healthier food to eat during emotional times. Choose food with a higher protein to lower carb ratio.

During long-term chronic stress, omega-3s can blunt the effects of high cortisol levels. In fact, many psychiatrists suggest taking omega-3s as part of antidepressant and antianxiety treatment. Omega-3 supplementation has been shown to reduce anxiety in healthy adults and is beneficial for persons with or without an anxiety disorder.

Omegas-3s have anti-inflammatory effects, assist in the formation of nerve tissue, and help receptor sites function properly, where important antidepressant and antianxiety neurotransmitters, such as serotonin and norepinephrine, work. You can obtain omega-3s through food or vitamin supplements, such as fish oils.

Food sources: Fish, especially tuna, herring, mackerel, salmon, and sardines; walnuts; and krill oils, which also contain the potent antioxidant astaxanthin

Magnesium is an essential mineral for health that is involved in more than three hundred biochemical processes. It plays an important role in helping cells make and keep energy and facilitates cell transport activities. A magnesium deficiency can lead to hyper-emotionality, generalized anxiety, and depression. In a group of elderly subjects, 500 mg of magnesium improved total sleep time, sleep quality, and sleep efficiency, according to a study published in 2012 in the *Journal of Research in Medicine Sciences*.

Food sources: Brown rice, wheat bran, pumpkin seeds, sesame seeds, almonds, and black beans

Tryptophan is an amino acid that enables your brain to produce the neurotransmitter serotonin, which becomes melatonin. Both are important for dealing with stress and promoting sleep.

Food sources: Chicken, turkey, milk, cheese, bananas, nuts, and sesame seeds

B vitamins decrease homocysteine levels, which become elevated during stress, depression, and anxiety. These vitamins help form neurotransmitters, such as serotonin, norepinephrine, and dopamine. Vitamin B foods and supplements augment mood, and a B vitamin deficiency contributes to depression and anxiety. Most importantly, B vitamins are required for almost every aspect of producing energy for our bodies from food sources.

Vitamin B food sources: Beef, pork, chicken, citrus fruits, rice, nuts, and eggs

B_1 *(thiamin) food sources:* Seeds, nuts, and pork

B_2 *(riboflavin) food sources:* Yogurt, cottage cheese, and liver

B_3 *(niacin) food sources:* Meat, wheat, and mushrooms

B_5 *(pantothenic acid) food sources:* Legumes, eggs, and yeast

B_6 *(pyridoxine) food sources:* Cereal grains, legumes, and leafy vegetables

B_7 *(biotin) food sources:* Cauliflower, peanuts, and mushrooms

B_9 *(folate) food sources:* Citrus fruits, leafy greens, and seeds

B_{12} *(cobalamin) food sources:* Salmon, cheese, and eggs

Vitamin E has a protective effect on memory and learning problems due to sleep deprivation and is required to inhibit inflammation of nerve tissue.

Food sources: Spinach, collard greens, beet greens, red pepper, sunflower seeds, pumpkin seeds, almonds, peanuts, nut butters, mango, and swordfish

High-quality proteins provide important building blocks for cells, hormones, bones, tissues, muscles, skin, and blood and should constitute about 20 percent of our daily intake of foods and liquids.

Food sources: Nuts, nut butters, beans, lentils, meats, cheese, eggs, yogurt, fish, and lean meats

Foods that Promote Calm

Fruits are good carbohydrates offering a variety of minerals and nutrients to replace those drained by stress. Also, because most fruits are high in fiber, sugar is released more slowly, avoiding sudden surges in insulin.

Vegetables also replenish vitamins, fiber, and minerals when you are in distress.

Foods to Avoid

You can have a nutritious approach to healing anxiety by changing a few eating habits. You may find this difficult if many of the foods you love are the ones that you need to eliminate. You deserve the best health, and changes that may seem hard at first become easier as you develop a routine.

Over time, stressors can cause chemical changes in your body. The changes affect your immune system and make your brain and body sensitive. Stress can trigger the production of inflammatory mediators that can lower your immune system's ability to fight off infection and leave you fatigued. In fact, psychological stress has been shown to increase the production of nuclear factor-kappa beta. Nuclear factor-kappa beta is a potent inflammatory producing protein complex that resides in our cells. When stimulated, it travels to the nucleus, where it turns on the inflammatory cascade. It functions appropriately when we are confronted by stressors such as infection or toxins. However, its unbridled production from chronic stress has been associated with many untoward results such as autoimmune disease, inflammatory bowel disease, coronary artery disease, and cancer.

Caffeine is a primary stress trigger and eliminating it goes a long way toward relieving anxiety. Coffee, tea, soda, and energy drinks/shots all contain caffeine. Some energy shots, for example, have levels of caffeine ranging from 200 to 500 milligrams. One cup of coffee contains caffeine from 40 to 100 milligrams, possibly more depending on the type of coffee. There are many good reasons to avoid developing a caffeine habit:

- Caffeine is a diuretic. It makes you urinate more, which contributes to dehydration.
- Caffeine inhibits serotonin in the brain, which triggers irritability and depression.
- Caffeine can keep you awake, and lack of sleep makes you stressed and anxious. It does this by blocking adenosine, a neurotransmitter that builds up the longer we are awake. Adenosine is a major factor in feeling sleepy.
- Caffeine does not mix well with some medications. When taken with Adderall, for example, it overworks the adrenal functions, causing more fatigue and irritability, and can cause insomnia, headaches, tremors, and an increased heart rate and blood pressure.

Magnesium is necessary for producing elements in the body that combat anxiety. Eating processed foods and drinking soft water, which lacks nutrients, and caffeine (which blocks the absorption of magnesium) can cause a deficiency and increase your anxiety. See page 92 for magnesium-rich foods to include in your diet.

Avoid foods and beverages with refined sugars. High-sugar products and foods that are high on the glycemic index can wreak havoc after the pancreas has released insulin to fight the sugar high. You will feel anxious and probably irritable after eating foods that are high in sugar because they lack nutritional benefits and cause digestion issues.

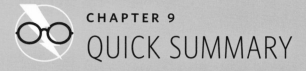

CHAPTER 9

QUICK SUMMARY

》 Manage emotional eating and focus on nutrients and supplements, especially B vitamins that support calm and health.

》 Incorporate foods to avoid and foods that calm in your stress management planning.

》 Change a few eating habits to better nutritious choices, such as adding high-quality proteins and reducing carbohydrates to foster energy and better metabolism.

Omega-6 fatty acids have become the predominant form of polyunsaturated fatty acid (PUFA) in the American diet. PUFAs cause inflammation. In fact, the ratio of omega-6 to omega-3 PUFAs in the American diet is now about 12:1. Most scientists believe this should be as it was hundreds of years ago, at about 2:1. Omega-3 and omega-6 work together, and you benefit the most if you keep a balanced ratio of omega-3 to omega-6. Otherwise, you may need to reduce omega-6 in your diet because an overload of omega-6 fatty acids is linked to moodiness, inflammation in the brain, and cardiovascular disease. If you eat poultry and eggs, which are high in omega-6, ensure that you also eat from the omega-3 food sources to balance the ratio, such as fatty fish, flaxseed, and chia seeds. Vegetable oils (such as peanut, sunflower, corn, and soybean oil) are also sources of omega-6s.

Changing your diet helps you manage your symptoms. Every step you take toward feeling better will give you the chance to explore other treatments as needed. Eat well and feel better.

CHAPTER 10

UNHEALTHY PATTERNS OF RUMINATING AND NEGATIVE THINKING

A primary characteristic of general anxiety is having unhealthy thoughts that are difficult to get rid of and repeat themselves. They distract you from everyday tasks. These can include negative thoughts about yourself, a situation, the future, or relationships. Your thoughts emanate from a critical voice in your head that feels it is helping you by warning you of dangers, failure, disappointment, and more. Negative thoughts often precede or accompany anxiety. Then they sustain anxiety and impair your sleep, leading to insomnia. That is when you practice skills of noticing feelings and reframing negative thoughts to stop the vicious cycle.

Put Your Feelings into Words

Have you felt relief when you spoke about your feelings with a pastor, friend, or life coach? Some people feel improvement when they can talk to others about their problems. Others intuitively know that naming their feelings or writing about their sadness, grief, or anxiety can lighten their load.

Putting feelings into words, called affect labeling, helps mediate negative, emotional experiences, but researchers wanted to know how this occurred in and affected the brain. When we talk about our emotions, brain imagery shows reduced activity in the amygdala and limbic system, which is the exact result you want for reducing hyperarousal. This suggests that putting feelings into words helps regulate negative experiences and diminishes hyperarousal and reactivity. This approach is ideal for people who tend to ruminate on negative thoughts.

What Is Rumination?

Rumination is like a compulsion to focus on distress, the causes, and any possible what-if events. Rumination is self-reflection gone wrong because the focus is on negative experiences. Rehashing the experiences alerts the defenses and agitates fears.

You may have heard a divorced adult repeatedly discuss an accusation or an action that took place years ago. A young adult may repeat stories of a traumatic car accident that happened when he

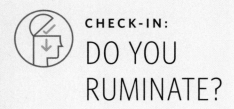

Rate each behavior on this three-point scale: 1 = never, 2 = sometimes, 3 = often. The higher your score, the more your mind ruminates. Do you think about or ask yourself:

Why am I being punished or why do I deserve this? ① ② ③

Why can't I just get away (flee) and consider why I feel this way all the time? ① ② ③

How did my problems become so hard to deal with and other people seem to handle them okay? ① ② ③

Why am I always reacting (e.g., complaining, blaming)? ① ② ③

Why am I not motivated anymore? ① ② ③

How will I be able to concentrate or focus if this feeling continues? ① ② ③

Why am I always so sad? I wish this were not my fault. ① ② ③

Did you notice that the statements of rumination are focused on self-blame and fixated on negativity? These types of ruminations are typical if you are in a hyperarousal state with an overactive amygdala.

was a child. If you have a similar pattern, your mind replays the words, scene, and fears. The emotional investment is so strong that you forcibly have to change your habits. Start with a checklist for identifying thought patterns associated with rumination.

It is amazing how putting it down in writing can offer a different, less emotionally charged viewpoint. People use various methods, such as medication, meditation, yoga, and exercise to reduce the sensitivities enhanced by hyperarousal. But the truest healing takes place when the brain and body can rest and repair. During sleep, much of the work you have done to stop automatic hyperarousal responses is consolidated.

Negative Self-Talk

Continuing to speak negatively or consistently making statements that are negative is another symptom of being in a hyperarousal or anxious emotional state. Chronic negative self-talk is like beating yourself down on a daily basis. Who can feel better and sleep better with this kind of stream of negativity?

Negative Self-Talk Patterns

There are patterns of negative self-talk, depending on the underlying emotion, whether it is anger, depression, or anxiety.

❯ An angry person may focus on someone's behavior to the exclusion of other qualities. For example, Karen, who was introduced in chapter 1, exhibited a chronic anger pattern due to insomnia, which caused her to dwell on her husband's care of their dog. Her memory became selective in how she thought and talked about his behavior. The pattern, similar to tunnel vision, is restrictive thinking, since the reality was very different. He properly cared for and trained the dog on a regular basis.

》 A depressed or sad person dwells on failures, problems, and situations that never improve.

》 An anxious or panicked person is always on hyper-alert for danger and anticipating the worst.

Other elements of negative self-talk are exaggerations, discounting, and self-deprecation. You may think that people feel sorry or negative because of you, or that nothing good happens to you. You may be deflecting your feelings on

someone else, or accusing another person of exhibiting behavior that is, in fact, more reflective of your behavior. At first, Karen accused her husband of treating their dog badly. At a later time, she admitted kicking the dog in anger.

Changing Negative Self-Talk

Healing hyperarousal and its manifestations take place through a deep sleep seven to nine hours per night. In the meantime, these six suggestions will help you to change the negative self-talk.

① **Become aware.** Examine your feelings and give them a voice. Naming your feeling—for

TO DO:
WRITE OUT AND DISCHARGE RUMINATIONS

① **Recognize it:** You start having that conversation with yourself about what you should have done or could have done, and it upsets you. Be aware of how you repeat the same conversation, story, or event over and over again in your mind.

◯ Recognizing that you are ruminating is a commitment, the first step in stopping this negative process.

② **Write it out:** Instead of having that repetitive, imaginary conversation in your mind, write it out. Write your words, your memories, or your rant in a letter or journal.

◯ Your first commitment to stop rumination is

to write down your thoughts until they stop. Patients report that writing pages of thoughts and feelings makes them feel better, as though they've released a heavy burden.

◯ Next, put the writing away and look at it the following day. What level of emotions rise? Have you discharged a significant portion of the rant? Are you feeling calmer now?

Find helpful writing prompts in Appendix D, page 150.

example, saying, "I am feeling anxious right now even though I do not know why"—helps decrease the level of anxiety you feel. Another variation of this strategy is to keep a whiteboard, small notepad, or an open document on your computer or phone in which you can write or type the negative thought. Then rewrite it as a positive statement and read the statement aloud.

② **Change your expression.** You can't stay in a negative frame of mind when you smile. Smiling is a powerful, transformative practice that your brain tracks. The more you smile, the more the brain monitors the positive pattern accordingly. Smiling releases tension, and cells relax.

③ **Sing to yourself and listen to music.** The effect of music can be uplifting for your mood. While listening to music, your perception of pain intensity changes.

④ **Move your body.** Shifting your focus at the physical level through dancing, walking, or running increases brain-derived neurotrophic factor (BDNF), which improves cognitive function and reduces anxiety.

⑤ **Step out of your comfortable space and help another person.** One of my patients, who developed acute insomnia after the death of a parent, chose to voluneer at the local humane society. She became a foster mom for dogs that were being re-homed and needed assurance, training, and tenderness.

With restorative sleep and animal friends, she changed her negative thinking and speech patterns.

⑥ **Pay attention to your body and change your stance.** Next time you are aware of your negative self-talk, take immediate notice: What is your body doing? Are you shaking your head? Are your neck muscles tense? Are you hunching over a computer? Stand up and shake out your tension. Then pose in a power stance (see illustration opposite). Try this power stance and hold it for two minutes. You will feel different, as if you are more centered or open.

Keep a Log to Change Negative Self-Talk

See the chart on page 102 and use it as a guide to creat a daily log to track and follow your negative thinking patterns. Review your conversations each day and write out any negative self-talk you experienced. When a pattern becomes clear, focus on changing that pattern for one week by choosing different words and thoughts that are more positive, upbeat, encouraging, and flexible. Continue to repeat those throughout your day. You can think, speak, or read the revised statements to ensure they become part of your new vocabulary. You are changing the language you heard as a child and teen that formed neural pathways, but you can form new pathways and achieve a different emotional state. Another way to change negative self-talk is to consider how to solve the problem. See suggestions in the chart on page 103.

Your ability to transform unhealthy thinking into positive affirmations is a powerful first step to feeling better. Next, to support the new neural pathways, you need to establish a sleep schedule of seven to nine hours each night to allow the brain and body time to consolidate new learning and memory. It is during this period that the emotional brain, amygdala, and higher cortical centers of our brains sort out thoughts, emotions, and memories. In fact, during REM sleep, when levels of the arousing neurotransmitter norepinephrine are low, replacing anxiety-charged memories with new ones occurs most efficiently. Experts in the field refer to this as "sleeping to forget." You will find that your memories are stronger and more positive with better quality sleep.

Schedule Time for Inspiration and Exercise

If left alone with your thoughts, what do you observe? Do you worry? Do you listen to negative newscasts? If you sit at a desk or computer throughout the day, how often do you schedule a stretch break?

One positive way to start your day is with self-reflection exercises or positive affirmations. Self-reflection might be a question that you ask and then answer as an affirmation. Schedule time in your day to support health, mindfulness, compassion, and calm. The following examples may spark new ideas. This exercise serves three important functions:

① It focuses your mind.

② It forces you to take positive action that relieves anxious feelings or apprehension. It shifts your mind to a positive emotional state, such as gratitude.

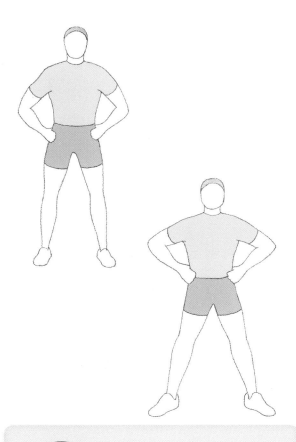

TERM REVIEW

Rumination is an obsessive focus on negative thinking and feelings.

Self-blame means turning the cause and reason back on yourself, which can detract from healing or motivation to change.

Lack of adaptive coping includes taking drugs, ruminating, or blaming or isolating yourself.

Change Negative Thoughts to Positive Statements

Negative self-talk pattern	Change to flexible, positive statements
Black or white: It must be this way or that way; there's no in between. "I can't see it that way. You agree with me or you don't."	"There are other options, and I'll list two here: _____."
Magnifying thinking: Making a mountain out of a molehill. "I can't ever call her because she is always cranky when I call, and I don't want to bother her again. I'm sure it is my fault."	"I enjoy talking with her. The truth is that I don't know why she is cranky, and I do not know whether her being cranky is my fault. The simple solution is to set up an appointment with her and call. I will ask her how she is feeling and whether if I've done something to upset her."
Minimizing: Focusing always on your mistakes and putting yourself down. "I notice you didn't eat the vegetables at dinner. I must have overcooked them. I'm not a good cook at all. I'm not even helpful in the kitchen. Do I have a bad attitude?"	"I notice that Jake didn't eat the vegetables at dinner. I won't blame myself. Instead, I'll ask Jake whether there is something wrong."
Always right: Needing to be perfect, to be right, to be heard, and to put blame or put others down for not being right. "You left the light on in the pantry. This is the second time this week. What is wrong with you? Why can't you remember? Do I have to follow you around and turn off the lights?"	"She left the light on again. I notice how that action bothers me. Rather than address her, I am going to put a sticky note on the door for both of us. The note will remind us to turn off the light when we close the pantry door. That way I will not come across as blaming."
Overly emotional: Your feelings are facts, and you believe only your feelings. "I feel so tired that I can't get this done today. Why am I so tired?"	"I can rest and then tackle the project." "I will take a walk and get past the fatigue."
Overgeneralizing: You always conclude that a negative event leads to bad things happening again or in the future. Your clues here are the words *always* and *never*. "We had such a great first date, but he hasn't called again. He'll probably never call me, and this will end like my other dates always end."	"The reality is that I do not know why he has not called me. What is the evidence that he'll never call me again?" "I can find out easily why he hasn't called. I can call him and find out how he is."
Inflexible thinking: Words such as *should*, *must*, *always*, and *have to* show inflexible thinking and rules that only exist in your perception. "I shouldn't go out right now. I should study, and then review materials for class. But I never get a break."	"What's realistic in this situation? Could I go out and also review materials for class? Am I setting myself up for failure if I don't review materials? I should estimate the time needed for the review, and then see if I have time to go out."
Blaming: Consistently blaming others or yourself due to anxiety or low self-esteem. "It is his fault that he stopped so quickly at the yellow light. I hit the back of his car by accident. When I saw that he wasn't going through the intersection, I slammed on my brakes."	"The reality is that I expected him to run the yellow light. I had to slam on my brakes, and I still bumped the back of his car. I can take the blame here."

Problem-Solving Affirmation

Self-reflection	Affirmation
What am I doing today to conquer anxiety?	I will start my day with twenty minutes on the treadmill while listening to music I enjoy.
How will I relax today?	I will get a gentle, relaxing massage. Or I will play nine holes of golf after work.
What will I relish about my life today as a positive action?	I will write one page in my gratitude journal. Or I will call a friend.

③ It helps you take charge and not feel helpless or victimized by anxiety.

You can also end your day with inspirational reading, calming music, or quietly affirming your wholeness and integrity by writing in a nightly journal. Such rituals help you relax and improve your ability to go to sleep and stay asleep.

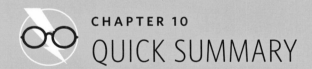

CHAPTER 10
QUICK SUMMARY

》 Thoughts that continually pass through your mind influence moods, energy levels, and how you interpret life.

》 Unhealthy or negative thoughts—part of distress, anxiety, panic, and insomnia—follow patterns associated with underlying emotions.

》 Negative thoughts fixate on self-blame and negativity and exacerbate hyperarousal symptoms.

》 You can stop unhealthy ruminations or transform them by putting feelings into words through writing. At the same time, this process diminishes hyperarousal. Start your day with inspiration and end your day with healthful sleep.

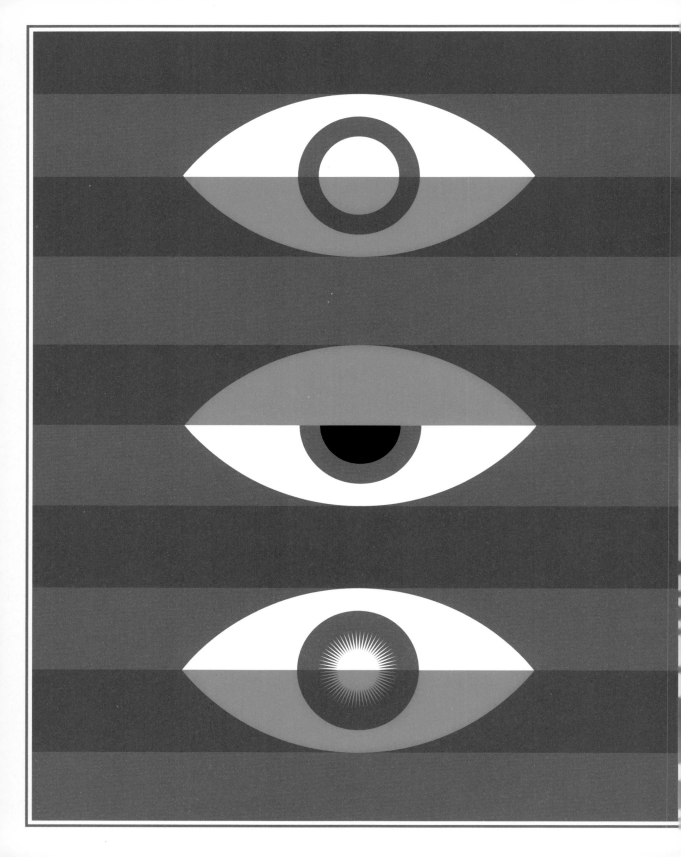

CHAPTER 11

THE LINKS AMONG GENERAL ANXIETY DISORDER, INSOMNIA, AND SLEEP APNEA

Although there are definite similarities, there are significant differences between everyday anxiety and an anxiety disorder. People with generalized anxiety disorder worry, and their exaggerated concerns appear not warranted or imminent. Their concerns could focus on most any issue, from health, finances, relationships, or work to current events or natural disasters.

A mental health professional diagnoses general anxiety disorder if excessive worry exceeds six months. During those six months, the person must experience somatic or physical symptoms for three months. Twice as many women as men experience a general anxiety disorder. The age of onset can be anywhere between childhood and the early forties.

While some people with a GAD diagnosis are aware of their behaviors or understand they exaggerate worries, they cannot seem to control their hyper-reactivity. They startle easily and cannot relax. They have trouble going to sleep and experience sleep disturbances when they do sleep. Their physical discomforts include tension, fatigue, headaches, nausea, dizziness, and trembling.

The length of time for the symptoms is key to the diagnosis. Once an anxiety pattern is set, your mind recreates the memory, and then you exhibit fear about the experience. The chart (page 106) clarifies the difference between anxiety you might experience on any day and general anxiety disorder.

These few examples illustrate the differences between constant anxiety and generalized anxiety disorder. People with mild anxiety can continue to work and socially function in relationships. Others with a severe level of

TERM REVIEW

Generalized anxiety disorder (GAD) is a prevalent, chronic, and debilitating mental illness that is associated with marked impairment in daily functioning.

Anxiety versus General Anxiety Disorder

Everyday anxiety	General anxiety disorder (GAD)
You are nervous or uncomfortable when in a large group of people you don't know, but you still can participate in the social function.	You avoid going out in public or being in social situations, because of fear of those interactions.
You are nervous about being in front of a group of people or your colleagues.	You experience panic attacks when you think about being on stage or addressing professionals at a business convention. You are worried about future panic attacks, resulting in further isolation.
You experience difficulty in concentrating and feel scattered.	You experience considerable difficulty in concentration and focus.
You experience difficulty remembering minor daily concerns or details.	You experience marked difficulty with memory.

generalized anxiety disorder have difficulty with daily tasks because of the mental irregularities of excessive thinking, ruminations, and constant what-if questions. Treatment for GAD and other anxiety disorders includes medication; psychotherapy, such as cognitive behavioral therapy; and lifestyle practices, such as mindfulness meditations, yoga, or daily exercise routines.

A Word about Medications

In recent decades, doctors have prescribed the following drug groups for anxiety, depression, and related disorders. Typical medications for anxiety disorders have included the SSRI group and the SNRI group. Speak with your physician about their use, risks, and efficacy.

SSRIs refer to selective serotonin reuptake inhibitors. SSRIs are typically used for the treatment of depression, obsessive-compulsive disorders, posttraumatic stress disorders, bulimia

nervosa, anxiety, and panic disorder. Serotonin occurs naturally in the body and functions as a neurotransmitter that transmits impulses across nerve synapses. In the brain, serotonin is found in the midbrain and the hypothalamus, regulating aggression, sleep, hunger, and moods. Thus, changes in the serotonin levels are associated with mood disorders. The amygdala is rich in serotonin receptors. Most serotonin in the brain is made in a brainstem structure called the median raphe, which projects numerous tendrils to areas of the brain that have serotonin receptors.

SNRIs refer to serotonin and norepinephrine inhibitors that are used to treat anxiety and depression. Patients with anxiety disorders frequently have insomnia. In fact, insomnia commonly occurs at the same time or quickly follows the anxiety disorder. A prescription for an anxiety medication depends on your doctor's preferences and your symptoms. Some types of medications that are used include antidepressants, benzodiazepines, beta-blockers, and buspirone, which is predominantly for anxiety and psychiatric disorders. Medications for anxiety do not cure the anxiety, but are meant to improve coping and functioning in daily life.

General anxiety disorder (GAD) is often responsive to antidepressants and benzodiazepines, such as alprazolam, diazepam, and lorazepam. Buspirone is a selective serotonin HT1 serotonin receptor agonist. It is unlike anything else available and is for anxiety only. The medications provide relief of the anxiety symptoms belonging to the motor and vigilance-scanning clusters. However, benzodiazepines are potentially addictive and are associated with an increased incidence of Alzheimer's (see more on page 74).

Common Causes of Sleep Disturbance

Health-care providers refer many patients with insomnia to sleep clinics. One such patient, Rebecca, despite taking medication, improving sleep habits, and trying psychotherapy, still has trouble falling or staying asleep.

Rebecca retired from a civil service job at the age of forty and moved closer to where her daughter was attending college. She was on medication for hypothyroidism (with test results within normal range), general anxiety disorder, and menopause. Though she had been taking antianxiety medication for eight years, she reported she was not sleeping or functioning better. Rebecca experienced problems staying asleep and occasionally falling asleep. She took copious notes in which she dexribed the following:

- Worrying often due to serving as caretaker for her father, who had dementia and later passed away. Even after his death, she reported a constant worry pattern focused on something bad happening.
- Going to bed at 10 p.m. and then listening to relaxing music or meditating for twenty minutes. Even when she fell asleep promptly, she would wake up within the hour, doze some more, and wake up again.
- Living with her college-age daughter, who reported hearing her mother snoring and being "jumpy" while she slept (constantly moving her legs).

Despite medication, Rebecca's GAD scores were still very high and indicated a continuing general anxiety disorder. We scheduled her for a sleep study to monitor her snoring.

I frequently find that my patients who suffer from anxiety or depression and are not responding to treatments have a coexisting sleep disorder, especially sleep apnea, which is at the root of their insomnia. Sleep apnea can damage structures in the limbic system associated with anxiety and depression. This manifestation of sleep apnea is more common in women than in men. It is no coincidence that these patients may have trouble staying asleep along with their anxiety or depression. In some cases, the sleep-related breathing disorder intensifies their anxiety. Although sleep apnea tests can be done at home now, I recommended a sleep study for Rebecca. Sure enough, we found that she had obstructive sleep apnea.

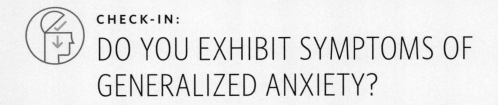

DO YOU EXHIBIT SYMPTOMS OF GENERALIZED ANXIETY?

If you are in an anxious state with hyperarousal, your worries do not go away on their own. It's important to catch the symptoms of anxiety early, so you can note their escalation and determine whether you need a medical specialist for sleep and treatment for anxiety. Use the following scenarios to identify your ability to notice the signs of being a worrier or an anxious person.

Scenario: You are taking a walk, a shower, or driving, and you notice that the same worry you had yesterday and last night pops up again. The worrisome thought hangs around and seems to be an intrusive presence. In fact, the more you try to ignore this worry, the louder and bolder it seems.

◯ Do you notice that you worry a lot? Do you worry about the same topic repeatedly?

Scenario: At work, you happen to overhear a coworker's rant about another employee. The rant sounds angry, and it triggers an anger response in you, too. That employee was rude to you, too. That rant continues in your head throughout the day.

◯ You follow a good schedule, but hyperarousal still exists. When your responses are angry, or they make you rant and worry, it is time to help yourself by using one writing strategy to put your thoughts into perspective. Moreover, start a sleep hygiene activity (see page 35) to ensure healthy sleep.

Scenario: You put the children to bed, take a long, hot shower, and crawl into a comfortable bed. The room is dark, even peaceful. You close your eyes to relax. You must have dozed off, because your body jumped, and now you are awake. You see that a whopping ten minutes have passed, but you thought it was morning. Now you're irritated. Maybe you punch the pillow, roll over, cover your head, and try again to sleep. This lack of sleep happened last night. And the night before. And the night before. No doubt it will happen again. Now you are awake.

◯ Does your complaining mind worry and keep you awake? Are you tense when you try to sleep? Then it is time to learn to relax through a peaceful meditation and hot cup of chamomile tea to help you sleep at night.

Scenario: Out of the blue, you feel a bit nervous or shaky, but you can manage it. Maybe you take several deep breaths or distract yourself successfully. At what point can you no longer distract yourself?

◯ Do you feel a flash of panic or anxiety often? Do you feel shaky, trembling, out of breath, or tired?

Scenario: You become overwhelmed at loads of laundry, a big work project, or starting a new college class. Your first inclination is to leave, ignore it, or forget about it until another time. But you catch yourself being overwhelmed, and you make yourself do a load of laundry or open the textbook. You handled that one!

○ Is your feeling of being overwhelmed increasing? Do you have trouble concentrating on one task or completing another task? Is it easier to distract yourself rather than face the pile of papers or dirty dishes? It is good that you notice. When you ignore and turn away from the list of stuff to do, talk it over with a friend. Review the sleep patterns and stressors in this book. Choose one strategy only and start to change.

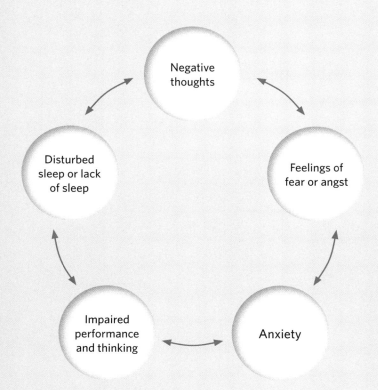

Unhealthy Thinking-Anxiety Cycle
The diagram shows how the cycle of hyperarousal can start with negative thinking or lack of sleep or anxiety. Once this cycle is activated, each activity reinforces the next and triggers the continuation of the cycle.

How Sleep Apnea Triggers Insomnia

Sleep apnea is related to the size of a person's upper airway. A sleeping patient is likely to have obstructed breathing and airway collapse if the airway is smaller in diameter. Conditions such as obesity, large tonsils, an enlarged tongue, or a backward-positioned jaw produce a smaller airway. Alcohol and certain medications further weaken the airway muscles when we sleep.

With sleep apnea, the sleeper's oxygen level drops. The sleeper awakes attempting to breathe against a closed airway. If this occurs repeatedly through the night, it can lead to insomnia. A sleep study can identify sleep apnea. Sleep apnea tends to be most severe during REM sleep, the very sleep you need to process emotions.

TERM REVIEW

Obstructive sleep apnea, or sleep apnea, is a sleep disorder characterized by repeated pauses in breathing throughout the night that disrupt sleep. Sleep apnea occurs when the upper airway briefly collapses during sleep. This results in drops in oxygen, elevated stress hormones such as adrenaline and cortisol, and triggering of the sympathetic nervous system. These episodes may occur as many as one hundred times per hour.

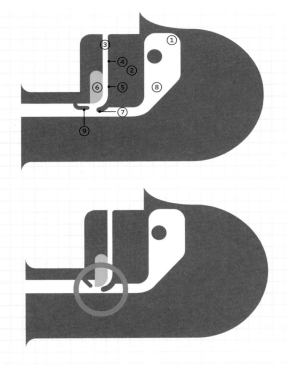

Sleep apnea

Sleep apnea is a sleep disorder that occurs when breathing is briefly and repeatedly obstructed during sleep.

① Nasal cavity   ⑥ Tongue

② Sinus cavity   ⑦ Uvula

③ Oral cavity   ⑧ Nasopharynx

④ Hard palate   ⑨ Epiglottis

⑤ Soft palate

Other Possible Triggers for Insomnia

Although this book focuses on the more common causes of insomnia, many others exist. Consult your physician if you suspect another cause, such as any of the following:

〉 Restless legs syndrome (RLS)
〉 Frequent urinating at night
〉 Leg cramps
〉 Nightmares
〉 Hot flashes
〉 Panic attacks
〉 Aches and pains due to fibromyalgia or low vitamin D
〉 Drops in oxygen due to pulmonary diseases such as chronic obstructive pulmonary disease (COPD)
〉 Central sleep apnea referred to as Cheyne-Stokes respiration due to cardiac disease

Several of these concerns are described in more detail in chapter 12. A health professional could ask that you participate in a sleep study to determine the cause of insomnia.

Treatment for Sleep Apnea

The most thoroughly researched treatment for obstructive sleep apnea is continuous positive airway pressure (CPAP) therapy. The CPAP machine pushes a constant stream of air through a mask that keeps the throat and airway open. There are different kinds of masks. Some fit over the nose. Others, called nasal pillow masks, fit into the nose while others fit over both the nose and the mouth. For effective treatment, the patient must use the machine every night, and possibly for the rest of his or her life. Patients can choose to cure their sleep apnea through some

WHAT HAPPENS DURING A SLEEP STUDY?

During a sleep study, a doctor analyzes your sleep by measuring brain waves, respiration, pulse, limb movements, and eye movements that characterize each stage of sleep. The doctor evaluates how you sleep and reviews your sleep patterns over time.

A sleep study takes place in a sleep center. The sleep professional will need a list of all medications, prescriptive and otherwise, as well as any substances you take. You prepare for sleeping at the center as you would at home. A sleep technician will apply the sensors and other monitors that register your responses. All of the monitoring paraphernalia are designed for comfort, length, and flexibility so as not to inhibit or disturb your sleep in any way. A sleep technician will monitor your sleep all night. The data from the sleep study is extensive, but the sleep doctor will interpret this and discuss any results with you.

other means (surgery or weight loss). However, after three months of consistent use, CPAP also restores the gray matter of the brain that was lost due to the sleep disorder. Within a year, much of the white matter damage, which involves the nerve tracts, also resolves for many patients. This treatment could also help general anxiety disorder by curing the sleep disorder that might be fueling the anxiety.

Sleep Apnea and Anxiety Disorder Links

Recent studies depict a high incidence of anxiety in people with obstructive sleep apnea (OSA), especially women. The reason may lie in the limbic system, a part of the brain that regulates autonomic and endocrine functions, particularly in response to emotional stimuli and physical threats. The limbic system contains the amygdala, which receives the information. This is passed on to the hippocampus, which compares the stimuli to prior memories. If it perceives information as foreign or threatening, the fight-or-flight activation of the sympathetic nervous system releases stress hormones. (See diagram on page 46.) This impairs one's ability to deal with stressors or severe psychological trauma associated with another anxiety disorder called post-traumatic stress disorder (PTSD).

During sleep, especially REM sleep, you emotionally reconcile the day's events. Sleep apnea severely fragments your sleep and hinders your ability to consolidate emotional events.Sleep apnea can thus lead to anxiety disorders in part due to interference with REM sleep, and in part due to structural damage as a result of low oxygen levels, high cortisol levels, and inflammation due to oxidative stress.

QUICK SUMMARY

》 People who experience generalized anxiety disorder (GAD) have difficulty functioning each day because of excessive thinking difficulties.

》 Excessive hyperarousal also involves sleep disturbances that could manifest as insomnia, sleep apnea, or other concerns.

》 Twice as many women as men are diagnosed with GAD. Symptoms include feeling overwhelmed; excessive worry; rumination; and difficulty with memory, focus, and concentration.

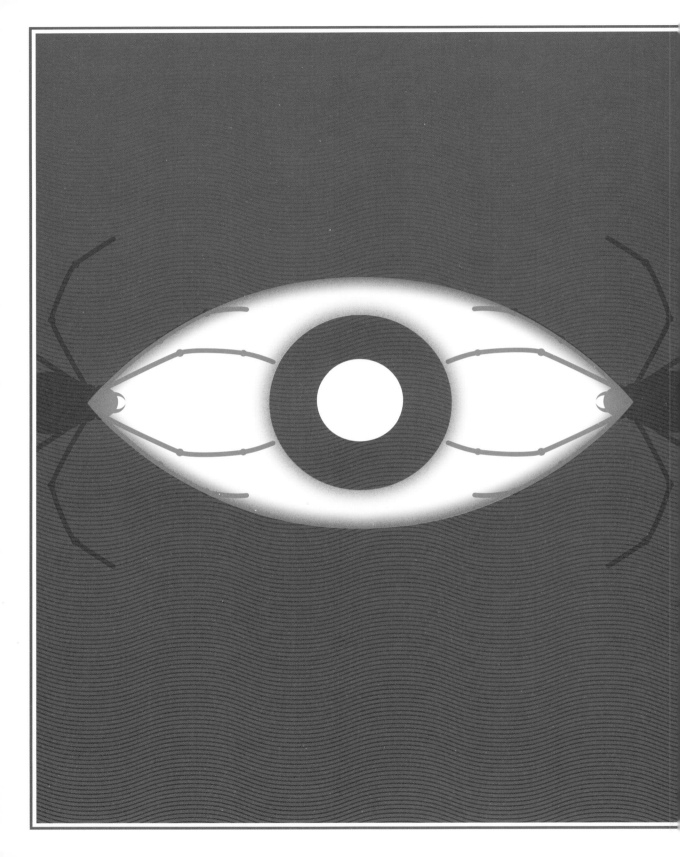

CHAPTER 12

OTHER SLEEP DISORDERS

Arange of sleep disorders, aside from insomnia and sleep apnea, are associated with or can contribute to distress, anxiety, or panic.

Nightmares

Have you experienced a dream that was frightening and provoked fear? If you woke up feeling distressed, scared, or anxious, you most likely felt relief upon waking and realizing that you had a nightmare. They occur mostly in the REM (rapid-eye-movement) stage of sleep that increases in the latter part of the night. Nightmares start in childhood usually before pubescence. Adults who have nightmares experience a vivid reality that can feel threatening. They recall the content clearly and do not go back to sleep quickly.

Although nightmares are more frequent in posttraumatic stress disorder, the conditions of anxiety, depression, and insomnia can cause isolated or recurring nightmares. Another cause of nightmare disorder that is frequently underdiagnosed is sleep apnea. Sleep apnea is particularly severe during dream sleep because paralyzed muscles and our brain allow oxygen levels to drop to the lowest levels. I have had countless patients with nightmares receive treatment for sleep apnea, and this reduced or eliminated their nightmares.

Another cause of nightmares that primary care physicians often overlook is the use of certain prescription drugs used to treat anxiety, panic, and depression. These include monoamine oxidase inhibitors (MAOIs), benzodiazepines, selective serotonin reuptake inhibitors (SSRIs), and serotonin and noradrenaline reuptake inhibitors (SNRIs), all of which can cause nightmares. Please note that you must consult with your physician before stopping a medication, even if you are experiencing nightmares. Some of these drugs can trigger withdrawal symptoms and must be managed closely by your doctor.

Ginger's Nightmares and Coping Strategies

Ginger was an overweight, twenty-two-year-old junior at the local university. She was a teaching assistant for the psychology department, in which one of the students conducted a sleep study as part of his research project. Part of the project involved taking a sleep survey. Ginger reported having frightening dreams at least twice per week, becoming routine within the last two months.

I asked Ginger about her course load and teaching work. She reported taking fifteen hours of coursework in psychology. She also worked three to five hours, five evenings per week, which involved lecturing, grading papers, writing, and research. She reported difficulty concentrating on work, making more errors than usual, and being tardy for class twice.

Prior to our appointment Ginger had kept a sleep diary for two weeks, as instructed. She reported having two types of nightmares. In one dream, she was chased by a wolf pack while hiking in a mountainous wilderness area. In another dream, spiders crawled up her bed, and she found her bed infested with them. These dreams were so vivid that she would wake up wired and stay alert afterward. She would turn the light on and try to calm down by reading or watching television. She admitted they did less to calm her down than distract her from her dream. She also reported that her mother often had horrible nightmares and was always anxious. Her mother had passed away seven months earlier from breast cancer. To make matters worse, when Ginger tried to fall back to sleep after a nightmare, she would ask herself, "Do I have insomnia? Did I inherit my mother's patterns of anxiety? Are these nightmares a sign of poor mental health?" Lastly, she noted that her roommate reported Ginger had a snoring problem.

My opinion was that there were three reasons for Ginger's nightmares. They seemed related to stress due to her coursework and teaching assistant duties. Her mother's death was a significant contributor, and she also worried about turning out like her. Ginger was clearly a bright student and a leader, causing her stress when she could not perform at her best. For Ginger, the nightmares were a warning sign. She paid attention to those warning signs and took action to get help.

My concern about the nightmares was her state of feeling wired, that she had to get out of bed and distract herself to quiet the anxious feelings. And it wasn't working.

The first place to start was with a sleep study to rule out sleep apnea. Ginger was overweight and snoring, two potential triggers for sleep apnea. Next, I offered her two sets of instructions, one on how to practice diaphragmatic breathing, which would help her relax, and the other on vitamin supplements for her to take, including food sources for those vitamins. I asked her to continue her sleep diary and begin a food diary.

Ginger was one of the 75 percent of young college women that develop anxiety and experience symptoms around age twenty-two. The consequences of her nightmares impaired daytime functioning based on Ginger's report. Her disrupted sleep and her compensating behaviors of working longer and harder were as annoying as her dream states.

Her coping skills were in keeping with her achievement-oriented personality. She persisted, worked hard, and kept moving forward. That pattern can wear down the adrenals, and her sleep disturbances exacerbated the hyperarousal pattern. However, beneath the professional demeanor, she still harbored grief, and her nightmares triggered fears of having more of them.

Fear is the most common emotion when waking up from a nightmare, and Ginger was fearful. However, she didn't demonstrate or convey anger, confusion, or guilt about her nightmares. Her primary fear was becoming like her mother's psychiatric profile, which included depression and daily medications. What more could Ginger learn about the nature of her fear as a child? What more would she reveal about her fear of turning into her mother now that she was an adult?

To cope better, Ginger developed compensatory behaviors, such as working harder, studying more, and excelling scholastically. That type of schedule did not leave much time to grieve her mom's death, take relaxation time, or hang out with friends now and then. When a parent dies, high levels of the brain neurotransmitter norepinephrine follow the emotional trauma and are a significant contributor to both daytime and nighttime problems. It causes hyperarousal and disrupts REM sleep, which is necessary for coping with emotional trauma and promoting the fear extinction process.

Ginger's sleep study revealed that she also had sleep apnea. I suggested a continuous positive airway pressure (CPAP) machine as the effective treatment solution. Treating Ginger's sleep apnea, which appears in higher than expected numbers for most trauma victims, decreased her sleep disruption and nightmares. Finally, I instructed Ginger in imagery rehearsal therapy, which is the most successful cognitive behavioral therapy for nightmares, to reframe and rewrite the nightmare scenario.

Imagery Rehearsal Therapy (IRT)

Imagery rehearsal therapy helps patients work through the content and feelings of a dream in a transformative way. The patient writes down the nightmarish dream, then changes the story to make it nonthreatening, and rehearses several times each day while awake. Through rewriting the narrative, a patient learns more about the

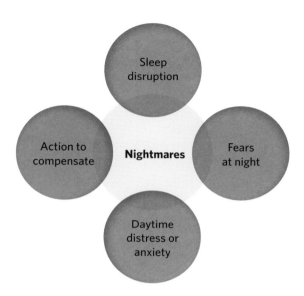

nightmare content, its meaning, and personal reactions. Ginger was able to recognize the intensity of her two dreams, as well as the imagery and the narrative. She reviewed how the content threatened her, what dream symbols like the spiders meant, and clarified more about her fears.

Although I am not a dream analyst, we did discuss what dreams about spiders could represent. In Ginger's case, they were coming out of her bed, possibly expressing a fear that was metaphorically swept under the bed and needs a review of content. Also, the stickiness of the web may be a metaphor for feeling entrapped.

I advised that Ginger keep a narrative diary about the time and frequency of her nightmares, if they continued. To desensitize her nightmare fears, she replaced the nightmare narrative with more desirable scenarios while awake. The result was to change a habit of dreaming by mentally rehearsing a new dream narrative and practicing it.

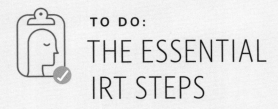

THE ESSENTIAL IRT STEPS

① **Identify dream content and discern why it does not work.** This exercise works best if you write out the nightmare. Writing as much detail as you remember, even though parts of the story are frightening, is helpful in gaining perspective and more control.

② **Identify a secondary narrative.** There are two ways to approach rewriting the script of a nightmare. If an entire dream featured scary scenes, you could rewrite the whole nightmare and create a calmer, happier story. If the ending of the nightmare was more prominent and fearful, then write a new conclusion. The new narrative triggers calm emotions and provides a positive image. The narrative should include positive emotions, such as hope, success, peace, laughter, or faith.

③ **Schedule at least twice-daily rehearsals and practices for at least five minutes.** You are practicing your new story with different images, and these should calm you and help you feel better. Your practice during the day prepares you for rehearsing the new narrative at night. After you are in bed and ready to sleep, rehearse the new dream right before going to sleep with no other interfering activities.

④ **Now relax.** After rehearsing the new story, practice a relaxation exercise such as meditation, hypnosis, progressive muscle relaxation, or deep breathing techniques.

⑤ **Keep a log of frequency, times, and your developing relationship with sleep and how you function during the day.** You'll be so happy to see your progress as you regain control of the subconscious fear that you brought into the light of day and faced head-on.

Continue practicing until the goal is accomplished!

Restless Legs Syndrome

Restless legs syndrome (RLS), a common sleep disorder, affects more women than men. The incidence of RLS increases with age. However, children also develop RLS, and people mistake the condition for growing pains. Health professionals consider RLS a disorder of the central nervous system related to the metabolism of the neurotransmitter dopamine. People with lower total body iron stores, measured by a blood test called ferritin, have a higher incidence of RLS. Iron is necessary for the formation of dopamine. Thus, medications successful in treating RLS stimulate brain areas that are receptive to dopamine. Normalizing ferritin levels with iron therapy can resolve the disorder in many patients. Characteristics of RLS include the following:

⟫ An overpowering need to move your extremities, usually your legs, because of an uncomfortable sensation that feels like itching, burning, or ants crawling on your skin. The movement brings temporary relief.

⟫ Difficulty falling or staying asleep. RLS, which occurs at night, is a major cause of insomnia.

- A genetic component. Forty to 90 percent of patients have a family history of the disorder.
- An association with low vitamin B_{12} and folic acid levels, as well as chronic renal disease, Parkinson's disease, fibromyalgia, and pregnancy.
- Often concurrent with depression, anxiety, and attention deficit hyperactive disorder (ADHD).

Health-care providers can treat RLS successfully. Low levels of iron and B_{12} are reversible. For people with RLS who do not have a particular cause, several excellent new medications are available. There is no reason to suffer from RLS when the possibility to reverse the condition exists.

Studies link a vitamin D deficiency to sleepiness and enlarged tonsils in children, resulting in pediatric sleep apnea. However, newer studies show that treating RLS patients by increasing the intake of vitamin D improves the condition, suggesting a link between RLS and vitamin D deficiency. A low level of vitamin D interferes with the function of an important brain neurotransmitter, dopamine, which controls the brain's reward center and helps regulate emotional responses and movements. We now know that dysfunction of dopamine is related to RLS.

Vitamin D is in fatty fish, such as mackerel, cod, salmon, and tuna, and in milk, cheese, and egg yolks. You can always use vitamin D supplements, as well as spend more time outdoors in the sun. In sunlight, your skin produces vitamin D. Risk factors that lead to low levels of vitamin D include dark skin pigmentation, limited sunlight exposure, living at northern latitudes, obesity, pregnancy, and abnormal intestinal absorption.

Some medications also reduce vitamin D, interfere with absorption, or accelerate the use of vitamin D, including the following:

- Antacids
- Calcium channel blockers
- A cholesterol-lowering drug called cholestyramine
- Phenobarbital or other anticonvulsant drugs
- Mineral oil
- Weight loss products that contain orlistat or olestra

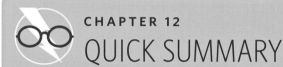

CHAPTER 12
QUICK SUMMARY

- Nightmares contribute to distress, anxiety, and panic. These hyperarousal conditions, in turn, can cause you to have nightmares.

- Sleep disorders such as restless legs syndrome and sleep apnea are also linked to nightmares.

- Treating sleep apnea frequently stops such bad dreams.

- Prescription drugs used for anxiety, depression, and panic trigger nightmares. Fear is the common emotion one feels when waking from these nightmares.

- A very effective treatment is image rehearsal therapy, one strategy from the cognitive behavioral therapies for insomnia.

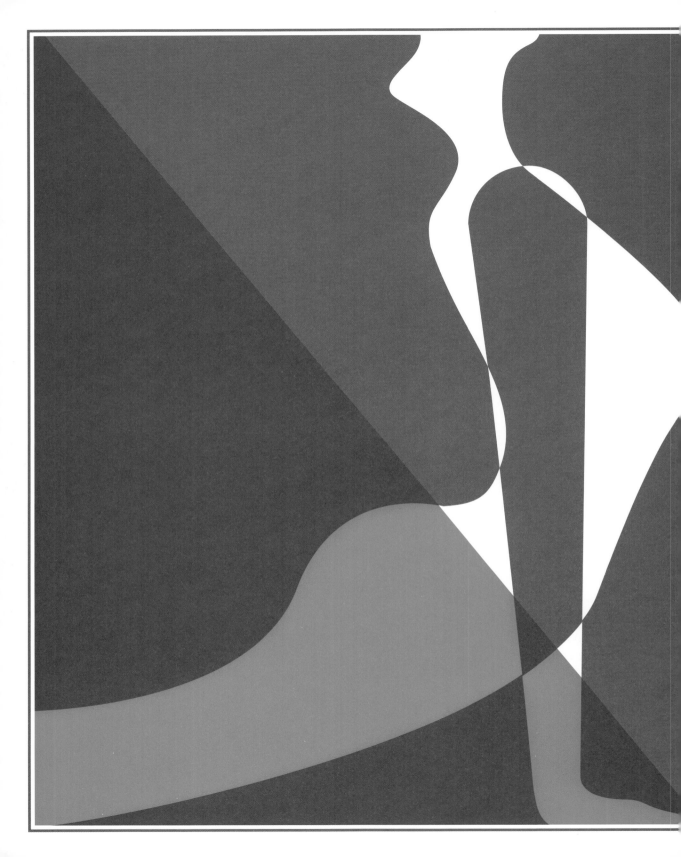

CHAPTER 13

PHYSICAL EXERCISES FOR CHANGING YOUR LIFESTYLE

Your lifestyle is how you choose to live your life every day, according to the values that are important to you. Your lifestyle reflects the following:

- Your interests, such as the movies you see
- Your routines, such as eating, sleeping, or working
- Your viewpoints and attitudes

Even the conversations you have with others reveal your character to them. For example, a high achiever might make this statement: "If it doesn't make me happy, make me better, or make me money, I don't make time for it." That adage sparks the image of a busy person focused on achieving specific life goals of wealth and happiness. This person is not frivolous.

As a sleep specialist, I see patients whose lifestyle habits and attitudes vary widely. There are three factors I've observed in patients' words and demeanors that convey to me whether or not they want to regain their health and will employ sleep medicine or other strategies that we agree are helpful.

① **Motivation is high to take action.** If you are sleep deprived, you will probably seek help because you are anxious and exhausted. Thus, you are highly motivated to take action.

② **Capability to act** is your speed and action in making better choices and changing bad habits. Will you take action? Or will you only *think* about taking action?

③ **Level of distress, discomfort, or pain.** Obviously, you will consult with doctors because these aspects are urgent. You want and need to sleep better, now.

Breathing Basics

The most basic movement of energy within the brain and body is your flow of oxygen through breathing. Most people breathe in a shallow pattern called chest breathing. This stressful breathing pattern is worse if you are overweight or obese due to the restriction of the diaphragm and airflow.

Breathing Basics

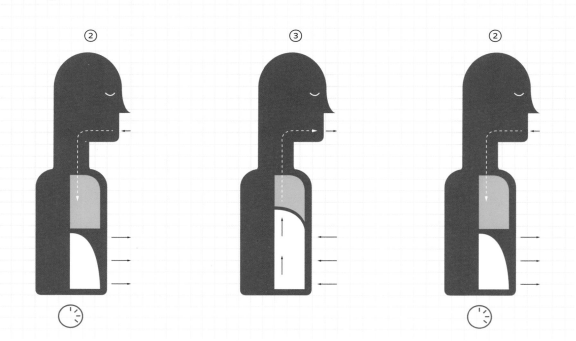

The first exercise, called deep abdominal breathing, is to breathe into the diaphragm area. This enhances metabolism, burns calories, and energizes you. Moreover, abdominal breathing triggers the relaxation response.

① Start and practice this exercise in a reclining or sitting position, so you feel the movement of your diaphragm. Close your eyes. Place one hand above the navel so you feel where to breathe.

② As you inhale slowly for four seconds, breathe into and expand the upper abdomen.

③ Now exhale naturally and relax. Then inhale slowly for four seconds and repeat.

④ Be still for a few minutes when you are finished. Let yourself fully relax. Allow your breathing to normalize before continuing with your activities.

Deep breathing is a safe and natural method that anyone can learn. It helps eliminate anxiety and hot flashes, is free and simple, and produces a more relaxed state of mind. To continue and expand this strategy, combine deep breathing with helpful guided imagery, which has been shown to enhance psychological wellness and reduce levels of anxiety and depression. For example, as you breathe comfortably with your eyes closed, imagine that the air you breathe in flows into your body and relaxes you. Imagine that the air leaving your body carries tension and anxiety away.

Full deep breathing deactivates the autonomic nervous system's stress response that instigates the release of adrenaline. It promotes a stronger immune system. In this next section, you can learn to use yoga postures along with deep breathing.

Practice Yoga for Relaxation and Pain Relief

If you have jet lag, stay up all night to study, or work in shifts, your circadian clocks are likely disrupted for a short time. You have to retrain your body's sleep patterns. Channeling your effort into a new habit through yoga is perfect and helps the brain and body relax.

Yoga may be the best option for experiencing positive health benefits, both physically and mentally. Practicing yoga increases your calmness and patience, which lowers your cortisol levels. Overall, you can expect to boost your mood if you practice yoga consistently. Exercise of this nature engages your body and releases your "feel good" hormones. When you take care of yourself physically, it transfers to other aspects of your being. If you have not experienced yoga before, know that it has wide-reaching effects on the mind and body by improving flexibility, joint strength, circulation, heart health, hormonal balance, and more.

Flexibility

Being flexible means bending easily without pain or discomfort. An obvious benefit when you practice yoga poses is a more flexible range of motions and less stiffness. By stretching your muscles, you release tension, relax joints, and energize your body and brain. Even five minutes of stretching once a day can provide you with significantly more energy.

Otherwise, tight muscles hold so much tension that you can strain your joints or end up in pain. Inflexible muscles, joints, and tendons shape into poor posture without strength. This derails self-confidence and leads to health issues.

Joint Strength and Stability

In yoga you move all of your joints through a full range of motion to stretch and strengthen them. This allows the joint cartilage to maintain its texture. It also prevents cartilage depletion from lack of use or exercise. Damaged joint cartilage can expose the underlying bone. Yoga strengthens without putting pressure on joints.

Better Circulation

Certain yoga poses such as warrior pose and downward-facing dog promote relaxation by increasing blood circulation to the hands and feet. Practicing key yoga poses can boost levels of hemoglobin and red blood cells, thus oxygenating tissues, tendons, and muscles. Increased circulation means you'll be less prone to blood clots.

Healthy Heart

Health specialists recommend yoga for optimal heart health. Using yoga to achieve cardio conditioning without the elevated heart rate can lower your risk of heart attack when you do yoga at least every other day for twenty minutes.

Lowered Cortisol Levels

Elevated levels of the stress hormone cortisol, which you experience in a prolonged hyperarousal state, affect your immune system and can lead to depression. Committing time each day to practice yoga can have a dramatic effect on cortisol levels, thereby aiding sleep.

Basic Yoga Asanas

Complete these basic asanas in sequence regularaly to maximize the benefits of yoga, including relaxation, pain relief, flexibility, joint strength, circulation, heart health, and hormonal balance, to name a few.

1. Relaxation
2. Eye exercises
3. Neck rolls
4. Leg lifts

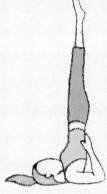

5. Shoulder stand (2 minutes)

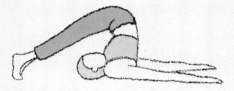

6. Plough (1 minute)

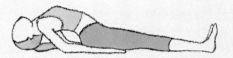

7. Fish (1 minute)

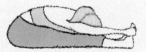

8. Forward bend (1 minute)

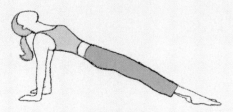

9. Inclined plane (30 seconds)

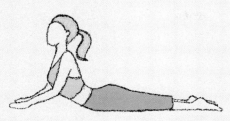

10. Cobra (2 times for 30 seconds)

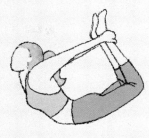

11. Bow (3 times for 15 seconds)

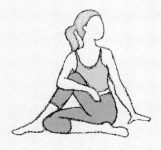

12. Spinal twist (30 seconds each side)

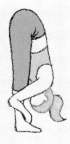

13. Standing head to knee (3 times for 15 seconds)

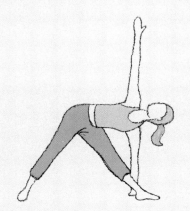

14. Triangle (15 seconds each side)

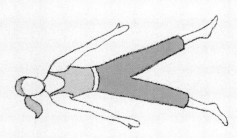

15. Final relaxation (10 minutes or more)]

Fight Fatigue and Stress

In a state of hyperarousal, you cannot relax. Your fatigue increases due to lack of sleep and relentless anxiety that drains more of your energy.

Participants in a recent study at the University of California (LA) practiced yoga for twelve minutes each day for eight weeks, and the result was a reduction in the immune system's inflammation response. There were lower levels of destructive inflammatory cytokines, especially IL-6. IL-6 is an important part of the body's inflammatory response and has been implicated in heart disease, stroke, and type 2 diabetes. Researchers also found the yoga practitioners had a decreased response to stress as compared to nonpractitioners. Other studies have shown decreases in pro-inflammatory IL-1 beta and cortisol and increases in anti-inflammatory IL-10 in yoga practitioners.

Results

Typically, yoga consists of three practices: a pose, controlled breathing, and a short period of meditation. The practices reduce the escalated stressors and are beneficial in managing anxiety, panic, and depression symptoms.

In a study of 200 breast cancer survivors, yoga was effectively able to lower fatigue by 57 percent and increase vitality by 12 percent. The women also showed between 13 and 20 percent lower levels of inflammation-related proteins compared with the control group. The improvements continued the longer they practiced yoga. The researchers attributed the dramatic results to the way yoga improves sleep through breathing and meditation, thus lowering inflammation.

Yoga Poses

Yoga poses (asanas) allow you to stretch and move your body in safe ways. They also help you shift mental focus toward healthy and positive thinking. Make a commitment to do this each day or at least every other day.

The poses on pages 124–125 begin with the basic movements, and each progressive exercise builds upon the previous pose. Each asana primes your muscles and organs for the next pose. Start with one pose at a time until you feel comfortable. Then add the second asana and so forth. You are building tolerance gradually and changing your neurobiology through each session. The practice of yoga is not hurried. As you perform each pose, do so slowly. Breathe, extend, and reach. This pace may be exactly what you need to reduce anxiety and stress.

If you prefer to have one routine that you complete at a comfortable pace, the Sun Salutation yoga flow (page 128) is perfect for you.

Get Fit

Exercising releases tension and has an overall calming effect for better coping with anxiety. Your lungs and heart breathe easier.

Getting fit means your sleep quality improves and normalizes blood pressure, blood sugar, and cholesterol levels. If you have thoughts about exercise being too hard or you feel overwhelmed about starting, then begin your transformative work on reframing your unhealthy thinking first. Then start imagining yourself with unbounded energy and resilience! Keep in mind that exercise is crucial for growing and maintaining healthy neurons (brain cells), not just growing muscle or losing weight.

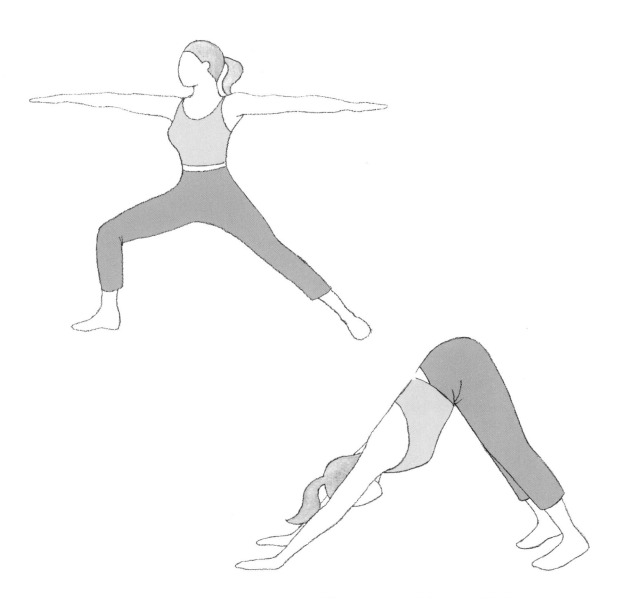

Warrior pose and downward facing dog
Increase blood circulation to your extremities thereby promoting relaxation. Practice these and other yoga poses every other day for at least twenty minutes.

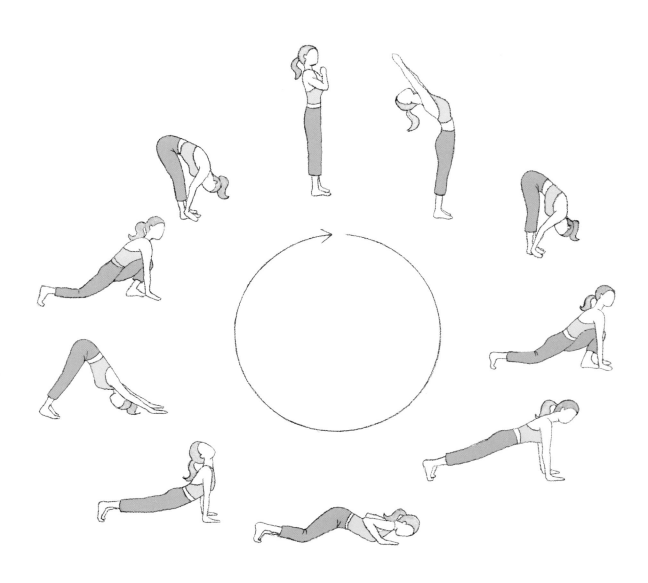

Sun Salutation sequence
Perform the Sun Salutation yoga flow routinely (every day or every other day) to reduce stress and anxiety.

People generally start out well when beginning to exercise for the first time or when starting again after an absence. However, one night of disturbed sleep or one stressful incident could throw you off balance. Or maybe you joined a gym or found a friend that would walk or play tennis with you on a regular basis. Then driving to the gym became a hassle. Maybe your friend bailed on you. When such small events happen, do you quit because it seems overwhelming? Now is the time to summon your inner strength and persist in making your decision to exercise happen.

When things appear to be going against you, that is the moment to persist. Stress and boredom will pull you away from your focus. Fatigue will convince you not to exert yourself. Your success depends on your ability to overcome these threats. Use positive self-talk and convince yourself that if you persist, you will accomplish your goals.

Set a Goal

Where are you headed? Do you want to gain or lose weight? Are you trying to become faster and stronger? It's important to do one thing at a time. Maybe you want to gain ten pounds of muscle and lose thirty pound of fat. Lose the fat first and then focus on gaining that muscle.

Ensure your goal has a deadline, as that creates a sense of urgency. A good deadline should be challenging but realistic. Write down your goal. Now create a loop for your goal (see below).

Make Exercise a Habit

You might think that exercise is a matter of only willpower. Willpower can help you persist in an exercise program, but it is a short-term solution. Exercise needs to become a habit, which is a behavior you build upon for solidifying a lifestyle pattern. When you dissect a habit, you'll notice that it is a loop that includes three elements: a trigger, a behavior, and a reward. When one of these elements is left out of the equation, the loop fails and the habit is broken.

Trigger. A trigger is a thought that occurs in your brain that tells you to take action. Usually sensory input, such as seeing, smelling, or touching, triggers a thought that tells you to do something.

To create a new habit, you must choose a trigger that serves as your call to action. Your trigger motivates you and exists in your everyday surroundings. For example, workout clothes, laid out the night before in the same place each time, is a trigger. You see the clothes, put them on, and go. If you have to search for them, it's not as meaningful and you will make an excuse to not go.

I still suggest that sleep is your first priority. Thus, placing a trigger on your nightstand forces you to review your decision to exercise every night and every morning.

Behavior. Your behavior comes from both the trigger and the motivation that you have for making the decision to exercise and committing to follow through. What motivates you?

- Would signing a contract of commitment to your exercise habit be enough to motivate you?
- If you signed a commitment contract in front of a friend or partner, would that help you honor your exercise goals? (Research shows that signing a commitment for a longer time frame rather than a shorter duration is more effective.)

> If you created a manifesto of your health goals and posted it in plain sight, would reviewing the value to your health motivate you?

Keeping your behavior pattern (habit) on track means that it will lead to something you're enthusiastic about. You may want to be in better shape for that thirty-year class reunion coming up. Asking yourself why you want to create the habit will help it stick. It will lead to the ultimate end of the loop that is the reward you'll get at the finish line.

Reward. New habits and old habits alike involve a reward at the end of the loop or path. Rewards are the satisfaction you get from a job well done, as well as satisfying cravings you might have. You want to be successful in your exercise program, so what reward will help you? A piece of clothing you've had your eye on? Meeting a friend for coffee? Reward yourself for your good behavior!

Create a Plan and a Schedule

If you exercise first thing in the morning, your evening will be free and you know you'll get your exercise done. However, most of us struggle to get up on time already. Consider using your lunch break for a little exercise. The evening has its advantages, too. Think about what will work for you. What time of day are you most energetic? What time of day do you need a break from more tedious activities?

> Night owls often like to exercise in the late afternoon and early evenings.
> Morning larks often enjoy exercising or running in the quiet of the early morning.
> Executives often schedule exercise routines during lunch hours.

Base your plan on your goal and deadline. Consider including a schedule, the exercises you'll perform, and the number of sets or repetitions. Your plan, like your deadline, should be reasonable. Avoid setting yourself up for failure.

Other Tips for Sticking to Your Routine

Finding a committed, experienced workout partner could be an important key to your success. Do you need accountability? Or are you self-motivated? Can you find someone that is as serious about working out as you are? Approach him or her and see if you can train together.

On days when you don't feel like exercising, do it anyway. On such days, you push through, and it feels fantastic! Those could be your best workout days. When it's time to exercise, it's time to exercise. The more you exercise, the stronger the habit becomes. You made a great decision, now work your plan enthusiastically.

Having a goal and a plan will strengthen your confidence. Seeing positive changes in your performance and appearance helps, too. If you do the right things every day, then success is inevitable. The energy you put into effort works well, as your brain and body will want more. Keep an image of wonderful benefits you'll gain by developing a strong exercise habit and keep it in your mind when the going gets tough.

You made a firm decision. This success will translate into other successes. All the variables are under your control. Put your best efforts into this first month to create your habit, and you'll find smooth sailing after that. In thirty days, you can have a strong exercise habit that will be resistant to change.

Remember this motto:
Healthy body, happy mind, healthy heart, happy life.

Remember this motto: Healthy body, happy mind, healthy heart, happy life. Make this your motto and memorize it. When you are tiring in the middle of a walk or treadmill exercise, say the motto aloud or in your head, and it will help you persevere, even if for five more minutes. It will be a good reminder for you to keep your body healthy and live a happier life.

For maintaining good health, only you will be responsible for now and forever. This is the main reason why you need fitness training to keep your body and brain in a healthy condition. If you fail to keep your health, you know the results.

Start your fitness with an active mode of exercise, as opposed to trying an activity such as meditation. Why? Anxiety makes you nervous and fidgety. Take the excess energy and focus it into a different activity such as walking, bowling, tennis, or taking a hike. Many people feel they have to go all or nothing. But exercise doesn't need to consist of hours of torture at the gym. Even taking a daily walk for thirty minutes can tremendously improve the health of your heart and the rest of your body. Or try another option:

》 Any active sport, such as golf, swimming, football, tennis, or basketball, is fun and provides good-quality aerobic exercise.

》 Include family members for a short biking excursion around the neighborhood.

》 If you really crave a unique, artful exercise, learn a new sport, like fencing. The art form is invigorating.

》 Dancing is yet another way to keep you fit and entertained. Put on music and start moving in your home or sign up for a dance class. The workouts are refreshing.

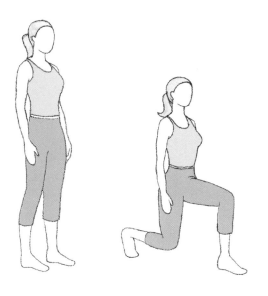

Lunge

Lunges, can be graceful, slow, and expressive. They work well as a core exercise because they use the core muscles of the abdomen, sides, pelvis, back, and buttocks. You receive the benefits of stretching, then holding tension, which energizes the core muscles of the body. It's important to maintain proper form so you do not strain muscles or joints.

- ⟩ Keep your back straight and relaxed, not arched.
- ⟩ Relax your shoulders and align them with your hips when standing.
- ⟩ Keep your chin up and stare straight ahead to focus on some spot in front of you, as opposed to looking down and facing down.

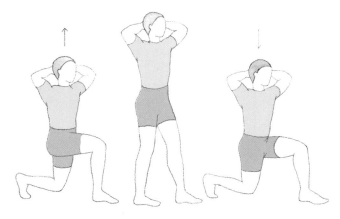

Bodyweight Lunge

- ⟩ Step one leg forward while lowering your hips. This will bend your knees. The front knee is aligned straight above your ankle. The other knee does not touch the ground, as illustrated in the diagram.
- ⟩ Balance your weight, and then move back to the starting position. Breathe deeply and rest.
- ⟩ Repeat and hold the tension of the lunge briefly to strengthen the muscles.

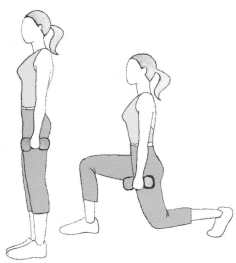

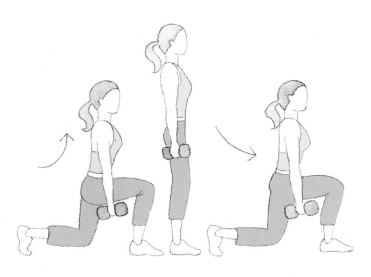

Lunge with Weights

》 Perform a lunge and add light hand weights of 2 or 3 pounds (1 to 2 kg). Hold them as noted in the diagram. As you feel stronger, you can increase the weights to 5, and then 10 pounds (3 to 5 kg). Holding or lifting the weights should not be strenuous or taxing.

Walking Lunge

》 Using weights, continue to walk forward, and then lunge. Alternate your feet with each step.

》 Lunge backward for extra conditioning only after you feel strengthened in the posture and proficient at lunging forward.

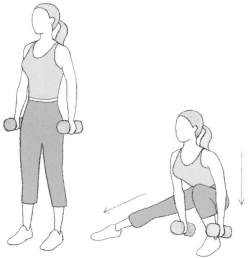

Lateral Lunge

》 While holding weights lunge sideways by stepping to the side and returning to center. Alternate sides with each step.

CHAPTER 13

QUICK SUMMARY

》 Physical exercise not only changes your lifestyle but also releases tension that builds up from hyperarousal and inactivity. Being physical starts a new lifestyle pattern for you!

》 Start with learning deep abdominal breathing that will come easily after a practice session or two.

》 You will feel different immediately and have more energy to start exercising for ten to twenty minutes each day. Will you choose walking, yoga, or lunges?

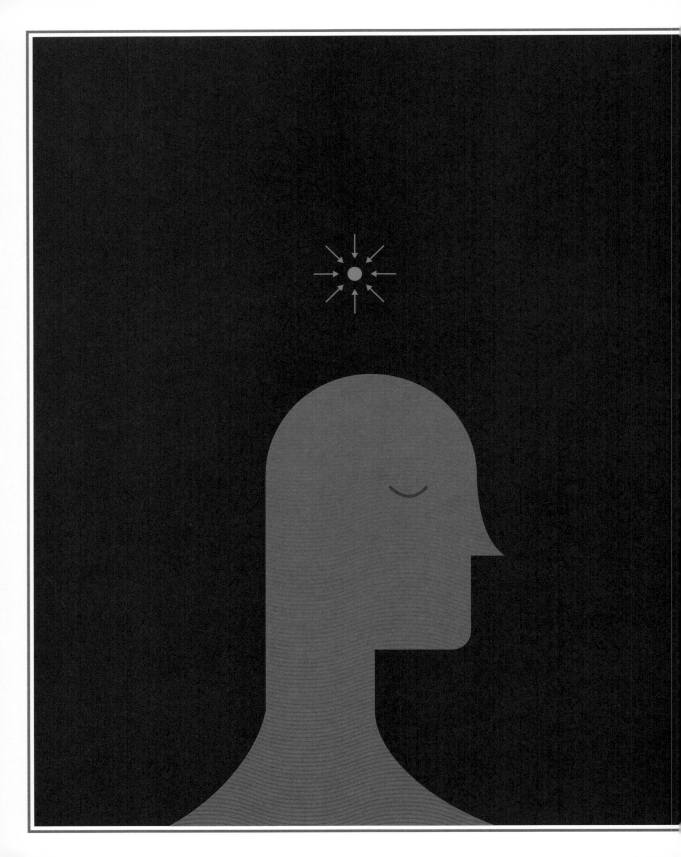

CHAPTER 14

MENTAL EXERCISES FOR CHANGING YOUR LIFESTYLE

A healthy lifestyle today involves a dedication to a whole way of life, embracing your thoughts and emotions in addition to physical health habits. Healthful living involves thinking, living, and acting as though you were preventing future illness or problems.

Focus next on the goals and the activities you need for healthier habits regarding sleep, stress-distress-anxiety, and nutrition. Consider an image or icon that symbolizes the lifestyle you want to achieve as you make your goals. Keep in mind your long-term plan to sleep and heal stressors through lifestyle changes. What are your goals? Write down your intentions. General goals are fine for now, as long as you know you can achieve them.

Good health choices can add up to thirty years to your life span. The most important lifestyle choices involve sleep, stress and anxiety management, and nutrition. Just thinking about where to start can be overwhelming, so I suggest that you start with sleep. If you do not have restorative sleep through which you experience the nighttime repairs, the quality of healing you need won't happen. Slow-wave sleep and REM sleep integrate learning and memory and balance the emotional biochemistry. Otherwise, you continue with the hyperarousal state, emotional overreactions, worry, anxiety, and sleep disturbances. The following mental exercises will help you change your lifestyle for the better.

Decide Rather than Choose

Making a decision on your first goal and designing follow-through actions is more effective than saying, "My choice is to start with proper nutrition." A final decision is a resolution. Think of a decision as your *best choice*.

TERM REVIEW

A **choice** is the power and the opportunity to select a path forward. A **decision** is the need to make up your mind, select the best path, and cut out extraneous noise.

By making a decision, you review the possible choices, eliminate options, and select a final position. For example, you decide to walk as your daily exercise. You wake up tomorrow, and it is muggy outside, and you choose not to walk. What does that reflect about you?

- ☽ That you make choices on a whim?
- ☽ That you dishonor your commitment to the "decision" to exercise?
- ☽ That you make choices based on external circumstances and not from inner strength?
- ☽ That you are choosing in the moment rather than following a decision that brings better results over time?

What is the difference between the choice and the decision? Think of your decision as confirming your resolve to do what is best. If you decide you will walk, then you walk tomorrow, and the next day, and the next, despite the weather.

A decision not to eat cookies for the next six months means you delete cookies from your food choices. You do not buy cookies or hide cookies in the kitchen cabinet just in case. The food no longer tempts you when you make a firm decision to exclude it.

Likewise, in reestablishing a healthy lifestyle, choices are no longer options. You'll need the competence to make solid decisions about sleep, first and foremost, as well as nutrition and exercise. Better eating and exercising are no longer options in your life. Rather, they are life-affirming decisions that demand your strength of will.

Meditation

Meditation practices are about consistently bringing your thoughts to a focal point within a set time frame. The focal point is determined by your goal and the type of meditation you feel will benefit your relaxation, sleep, nutrition, and goals. Your focus in meditations could be as follows:

- ☽ To empty your thoughts and float in space while you relax
- ☽ To repeat a phrase or mantra in your mind
- ☽ To put your attention on an image such as a pastoral scene that relaxes you
- ☽ To ask a question and be mindful of your thoughts and feelings for an answer.

Guided meditation, as in guided imagery, is when you enter into a meditative space by listening to a speaker lead you into a relaxed state. It is like taking an auditory journey. Meditation requires practice. Eventually, your mind will learn to rest. You'll be aware during meditation of how your breathing slows down and your blood pressure is reduced. Other benefits include the following:

- ☽ Relaxed muscles
- ☽ Less irritability and moodiness
- ☽ Elimination of lactic acid
- ☽ Clarity in thinking
- ☽ Reduced anxiety

A review of meditation's role in regulating sleep summarizes thirty years of research. The findings indicate that meditation regulates neurobiological functions in accordance with sleep. The earliest research on sleep and meditation involved practitioners of Transcendental Meditation. The focus was on a mantra and the purpose was inner peace and wellness. Studies showed the practitioners' physiologic state to be deep restfulness.

Another type of meditation, Vipassana, a mindfulness meditation that involves being aware of physical and mental phenomena, was linked to changes in sleep architecture. Meditators show enhanced slow-wave sleep and REM sleep. Further positive effects are regulation of the HPA axis and lower levels of cortisol and catecholamine. Research supports the idea that regular meditation alters the physiological functions in a similar fashion to what occurs in a sleep state. Meditation practices can calm your anxiety, decrease hyperarousal states, and promote better sleep.

Improve Your Sleep through Meditation

Meditation could help you go to sleep quicker and improve the quality of your sleep. In summary, meditative movements, deeper breathing, and meditations that make you relax are viable choices to manage stress and anxiety. Try these seven techniques:

① Breathe into the diaphragm and abdomen to release tension and relax.

② Cultivate the habit of listening to your body once you're relaxed. Starting at the crown of your head, scan your body and feel out any aches, pains, or discomfort. Notice the feeling. Use this time to relax more deeply.

③ Become more aware and mindful in the current moment when you feel tense. Notice the root of distress before it escalates and then breathe through that moment.

④ Multitasking erodes your concentration and builds up stress that may contribute to a sleep disorder. Multitasking stresses the nervous system and confuses the brain. Focus on one task and complete it before going to sleep. Get that task off your mind.

⑤ Discard judgments. You don't need unhealthy thoughts. Meditate before sleeping to empty the mind and open to space, air, sky, imagery, and relaxation. Meditation helps develop a mind free from judgment. Learn to look at your thoughts and cut back negative self-talk.

⑥ Use tai chi as a mental discipline by being present and conscious in coordinating slow movement with the breath. The art of deliberately paced, lightweight movements encourages deep breathing, stress reduction, and enhanced concentration.

⑦ Yoga refers to the unity of the body and mind and unity of the mind and soul. You've previously read about the health benefits of yoga practices. Built into each yoga pose is also a meditative moment or practice, depending upon the yogic tradition.

Decrease the Negative

Some activities move you away from anxiety-ridden moods by shifting your attention or removing the activities and triggers that magnify problems. Replace them with activities that bring enjoyment, make you feel cheerful, and most of all, help you sleep.

Turn off the television. Watching the news and reality shows overloads your sensitivities with what is not good in the world. Watching others suffer stirs up feelings that compound anxiety issues. If fear-based anxiety is an issue, watching events that make you fearful just exacerbates the problem. Those events trigger worry that what you are seeing will happen to you or someone you love. If you do watch television, choose lighthearted comedies that make you smile, informative shows, or those with complicated plots that intrigue your mind.

Turn off your electronic devices. Much like the television, these computer devices provide too much information. When you are away from television and other electronics, resist the temptation to take a quick peek at what's going on in the world. If you are prone to anxiety, leave your information gathering to a trusted friend or family member. Ask that person to contact you on a need-to-know basis if something important occurs. Of course, you want to be informed. However, the constant bombardment of information can be overwhelming. Do not sit with your eyes glued to the screen.

Increase the Positive

The simplest activities can be the most valuable tool for reducing anxiety.

Keep a gratitude journal. This helps you focus on the positive things in your life. Each day, record a few items for which you are grateful. Take several minutes to yourself to relax and soak in the positive things in your day. If you have a situation that has turned around for the better, be grateful for this transition. Make a note in the gratitude journal.

Take a nature break. Stanford researchers have shown how having a nature experience decreased worry and rumination and increased thinking and memory.

Take a walk. Or take a walk with a group, which can lead to even better results. Group walks have been linked to decreased depression, reduced perceived stress, and enhanced mental well-being.

Spend time with positive people. Simple distraction from your worries is one of the best ways to take a break. Being with optimistic people changes your focus, can change your viewpoint, and helps you put worries aside.

Get a pet. A pet provides much-needed stress relief. Pets help brighten moods and lessen depression. Playing with a pet increases levels of serotonin in the brain, delivering a calming and relaxing effect. There are even studies that show heart attack patients who have pets survive longer, and pet owners who walk their dogs regularly have improved physical capacity.

Stay physically and mentally active. Sitting around doing nothing turns the focus to worry patterns. When the mind is not focused, the door is open to rumination or anxiety. Close that door by focusing the mind and being active, because an active body releases endorphins that calm the brain and produce happy feelings and thoughts. Physical activity also improves general health, making you less prone to worry. Mental activity keeps the brain focused and improves the thought process, helping straighten out those spiraling negative messages. You can walk, swim, read, write, sing, or dance. Do something every day to keep your body and mind active.

> "In a world of high-tech medical gadgetry and space-age technology, the best software in the world is still that gray matter between your ears."
>
> —James S. Gordon, MD, author of *Manifesto for a New Medicine*

Volunteer. Volunteering is one of the most helpful actions you can take to lessen the effects of anxiety and stress. Not only does volunteering provide a fresh focus, but it also gives you a real perspective of your own life. You may end up feeling grateful for what you have, for what you can do, and for the people around you. You find the world is much larger than your personal experience, and people are genuinely appreciative of your efforts. The appreciation highly influences your self-esteem and moves you toward healing your anxiety.

Have faith. Living in constant fear causes anxiety because you feel you are doomed, either by external forces or by internal forces. Rather than live in fear, try living in faith.

Plan something to look forward to. Everyone needs something to look forward to, such as a vacation. Take pleasure in the planning and look forward to whatever the event is.

Practice positivity. Express your positive intentions through meditation, prayer, visualizing, exercising, or letter writing. Call a friend if talking changes your perspective to a lighter, brighter view. Do something positive for someone else. Also engage in positive self-talk. Say to yourself:

"Things do get better. I will have good days. Bad days don't erase the good ones. Good and bad days are normal, and I can handle it. I deal with life well. I am willing to change." The whole purpose of the positive activity is to activate optimistic thoughts and gain a new perspective.

Improve your environment and routine. Make small changes. You can start right now. Will you add more calming B vitamins to your morning routine? Will you take an evening walk? Can you call a friend that you haven't heard from in a while? Make one small change right now. Make another tomorrow. See what works best to relieve your anxiety. You will be pleasantly surprised to find a whole new world awaits you.

Begin a new hobby or resurrect an old one. Choose a hobby that uplifts you and doesn't bring on more stress. For example, you may have liked to golf at one time. But, golfing takes time and money. If these issues cause stress in your life now, perhaps a less time-consuming or less expensive hobby is better for you. Even simple tasks make a difference, such as doing puzzles, writing, gardening, or joining a weekly group for Bunko/game night or card games. Will you allow yourself some time to start and enjoy a new hobby? When you start a hobby, take a close inventory of your stress levels every day. Open your mind and see what else is out there.

Visualization

Visualization and imagery techniques are effective activities that relax the body and regulate stressors. Olympic athletes, musicians, and cancer patients have used the approach successfully for their goals.

James Gordon, M.D., author of *Manifesto for a New Medicine*, distinguishes the difference between visualization and the use of imagery. Visualization focuses on images. Imagery involves activating your senses, such as smell, touch, and taste, while you visualize.

A helpful way to understand visualization is to consider it a mental rehearsal of excellence. Visualization done well engages emotions and thoughts, which add a powerful element to motivate you to continue practicing. Emotions also play a major role in psyching yourself up to face and conquer anxiety.

Three types of imagery journeys are useful for stress, anxiety, and panic.

① **Instructional:** You start guided imagery with relaxation instructions designed to calm the brain and body. You can create your own or listen to a professionally produced guided script.

② **Feelings of safety:** Creating a safe place mentally serves as your retreat. You create a mental escape hatch to use during anxiety or fearful states. Images of pastoral scenes and waterfalls are calming. Imagery of floating among the stars can help you feel free and less tangled in emotions. If you need to feel connected, then imagery of towering redwoods can help you feel firmly rooted.

③ **Visualizing positive outcomes:** This is similar to designing a presentation of images that tell your story of how you successfully retrained your sleep and overcame your anxious thoughts. As you reflect on how you want to design a visualization journey, you can create a powerful mental picture of what the big prize will be. Then, you summon these images on a regular basis. Devote two ten-minute sessions each day or evening to remind yourself what you are working toward and why it is all worth it.

To start the visualization, find a calm place and state your intention: "I am de-stressing. I am going to relax and feel centered and calm."

As you center on your breathing, focus on your chosen image. Use as many senses as you can employ. For example, say you want to visualize a landscape that calms you. Picture yourself standing on a huge rock ledge from which you view this vista: an immense green valley situated in a canyon. You hear a rushing torrent of water, but can only see a snake-like path of a river far below. You see yourself hiking up the mountain, and you are almost at the crest. How does the backpack feel moving up and down with each step? How fragrant are the tall pines? Is the crisp air so full of cool freshness that your nose tingles? If your mouth is dry, taste the cool water on your tongue and lips.

Next, observe how you feel in your body. Is your breathing deeper or more relaxed? Do you feel tension release from your neck, arms, and abdomen? Are you calmer?

This visualization can be done at night before you go to sleep. To have a successful outcome, as you design the images for the journey, be specific when you define the goal for the images. Water images such as a tranquil pond can help you visualize calm. Ocean waves or a tall waterfall convey gentleness through movement and sound. Trust in your mental movies. The mind and body do not distinguish whether the visualization is happening in a physical way or in a mental way. To your consciousness, the event is taking place.

Another type of visualization directs the activity within your body. At first, you may see no images. As your mental instruction works, and you become progressively relaxed, the images form.

One of my patients used an exercise called "Turn on the Lights" (page 142) to relax before going to sleep. The goal is to imagine turning on a series of small dots of light. The sequence starts in your right big toe and moves upward to your knee joint and then your hip joint. Move the dots of light in three points along your spine to the base of your neck and then activate one at the top of your head. From there move to your forehead and down the front of your body, activating the endocrine gland at each center. Continue turning on dots of light through your left leg. This relaxing visualization directs your mental activity so worry thoughts don't intrude.

Yet another method is to visualize positive events from your past. By doing this, your brain and body will produce the feel-good chemicals to lift your mood and help you relax. If you don't possess a strong visual memory, just go with the feeling of wellness created by happy memories.

1. Think about a time when you felt happy and fully alive. It could be a memory of a carefree vacation or a time when you did not feel under pressure. Looking through your photograph album or reading through your journal is a good way to rediscover happy memories.

2. Once you've identified a vivid, positive memory, use your imagination to visualize and enhance the colors, physical sensations, sounds, and smells. Pay attention to how you look, what you're doing, and what emotions you're feeling. If these pictures are hard to visualize, just dwell in the joy of your pleasant memory.

3. Stay with this image or feeling for at least five minutes. Remember to focus on the physical sensations as well as the emotions.

4. Travel six months into the future and see yourself enjoying life and being happy and fulfilled. You have left your emotional difficulties behind. Look at your eyes, face, and posture. How does the future, happy you appear?

5. Travel even further into the future and see an even more relaxed, stress-free you. How does the future happier you seem now?

6. You can recall the feelings of well-being and contentment any time. See yourself smiling. You have left your stress and anxiety behind.

Visualization to Calm the Mind

Complete this visualization exercise (called "Turn on the Lights") to relax before going to sleep. Imagine turning on a series of small dots of light. Beginning in the right big toe upward to the top of your head, then down the front of the body to the other left foot. This exercise directs your mental activity, so worrying thoughts don't intrude.

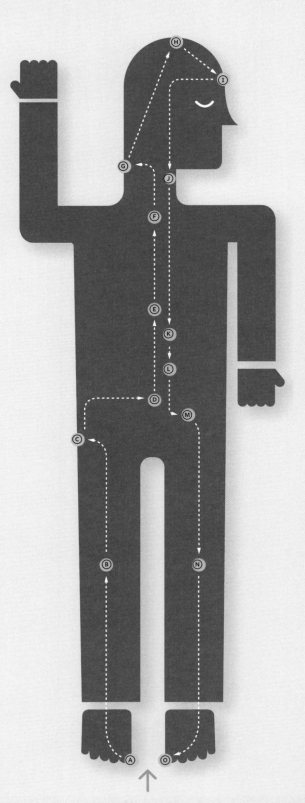

(A) Right big toe (start)
(B) Right knee joint
(C) Right hip joint
(D) Lower spine
(E) Middle spine
(F) Top of spine
(G) Base of neck
(H) Top of head
(I) Forehead
(J) Thyroid gland
(K) Adrenal gland
(L) Pancreas
(M) Left ovary
(N) Left knee joint
(O) Left big toe

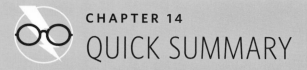

CHAPTER 14

QUICK SUMMARY

❯ Decide now to strengthen your mental resilience.

❯ Meditation techniques help you focus your mind on positive outcomes while relaxing your brain and body, especially before you go to sleep, and end your day with calm.

❯ Listening to your body's signals encourages you to notice what irritates your nerves or fatigues your brain so you can stop those behaviors.

❯ Replacing negative activities or stimuli with positive activity and calming environments will benefit your health, attitudes, and actions.

BREAKING FREE OF STRESS AND ANXIETY

Have no doubt that taking back control of stressors is worth all of your effort. Managing distress and anxiety breaks you free of the associated negative emotions that strangle you.

In this final section, I'll help you get the inside tension out through the medium of physically writing with a pen (or another instrument) in hand. I know many people prefer to type on the computer or dictate into an electronic device. However, the act of writing is therapeutic in reducing stress and increasing lymphocyte response, which suggests healthier immune function. Writing narratives frees you of inhibitions about the events surrounding stress, tension, anxiety, or panic.

The following suggestions for writing activities will get you started with positively oriented topics. The purpose is to help you clarify how you physically feel and link that to your emotional state or your thoughts.

Daily Check-In

Go through the list of negative emotions below at the end of each day. Note your feelings and physical reactions by placing a check mark by the words. Maintain this journal for at least a month to gain better insight. Remember that all of the following activities help you focus, shift emotional states, and diffuse tension. Remind yourself: I am a positive person with a purpose.

This chart helps you identify feelings for the goal of shifting to a different mood, if necessary, for your well-being. Ask yourself the following:

◗ What emotion am I experiencing?
◗ What physical symptoms do I feel?
◗ What triggered this emotion?
◗ How will I shift to more positive qualities?

Today I Feel . . .

◯ Hopeless	◯ Sad
◯ Depressed	◯ Angry
◯ Annoyed	◯ Anxious
◯ Vengeful	◯ Frustrated
◯ Disappointed	◯ Resentful
◯ Afraid	◯ Guilty
◯ Ashamed	◯ Envious
◯ Lonely	◯ Jealous
◯ Disgusted	◯ Hurt

Track Your Positive Qualities

- ○ Kind
- ○ Empathetic
- ○ Creative
- ○ Organized
- ○ Funny
- ○ Fearless
- ○ Committed
- ○ Patient
- ○ Confident
- ○ Playful

- ○ Resilient
- ○ Educated
- ○ Willing
- ○ Logical
- ○ Punctual
- ○ Intentional
- ○ Generous
- ○ Responsible
- ○ Loving
- ○ Logical

- ○ Trustworthy
- ○ Honest
- ○ Efficient
- ○ Supportive
- ○ Reliable
- ○ Adaptable
- ○ Flexible
- ○ Polite
- ○ Optimistic
- ○ Practical

- ○ Versatile
- ○ Takes action
- ○ Open-minded
- ○ Resourceful
- ○ Assertive
- ○ Charismatic
- ○ Loyal
- ○ Nurturing
- ○ Skillful
- ○ Trusting

To maintain a balanced viewpoint, consider your positive traits, too. You have the courage to see who you are and embrace the changes as you heal the stressors and anxieties. Make a list of your positive traits that make you feel good about yourself.

Reflect on Meaningful Moments

No matter where you are, you have the ability to feel peaceful and refreshed. A refreshing sleep of seven to nine hours is the priority. Getting back to nature is a second priority. When nature surrounds you, you feel peaceful and rejuvenated. If you can't get to a natural spot when you're upset, remember that you have the power of visualization to relax you whenever you choose. Visualize hiking through the redwoods. Let this feeling envelop you and drive the blues away.

Make a list of the places where you've experienced peace and rejuvenation. Then, you can journey to one enjoyable place in your mind. They'll always be there for you.

Find writing prompts on pages 150–153. Daily exercises such as these remind you of your goals to sleep better and feel fantastic. This book has brought you actionable strategies that you can use to sleep well and reduce the stress and anxiety in your life. The best plan is to implement these tips, step by step. Learn which techniques work the best for you. Soon they will become automatic habits.

However, the silver bullet of all actionable steps is to retrain your sleeping habits and learn to sleep well every single night. You will be making a serious mistake if you dismiss "a little

"The difference between great people and everyone else is that great people create their lives actively, while everyone else is created by their lives, passively waiting to see where life takes them next. The difference between the two is the difference between living fully and just existing."

—Michael E. Gerber, author of the *New York Times* best-selling book, *The E-Myth Revisited: Join the Entrepreneurial Revolution!*

sleep" as not important. These twin factors of not enough sleep and poor stress response are at play in your life if you experience even one of these symptoms: fatigue, obsessive thoughts, illness, poor focus, anxiety, brain fog, or lack of recall. Most likely you experience three or four of these symptoms that caused you to read this book.

Now you have answers for stress and anxiety symptoms. Now you have strategies to retrain sleep hygiene and allow your brain and body to restore you to health.

Sufficient, quality sleep is the single most important step you can put in place to offset and heal the stress-tension-anxiety-panic states. Sleep recharges your energy levels and amplifies positive moods. Believe it! Sufficient, quality sleep can solve the issues addressed in this book. Sleep well, be well, and stay inspired.

APPENDIX A

This checklist is also available for download and use from the Centers for Disease Control and Prevention at www.cdc.gov/reproductivehealth/Depression/PDFs/PPDChecklist.pdf.

The following checklist will help you start a conversation with your provider. Check the boxes that best describe your experience over the **past two weeks** and take the checklist with you to give to your provider at your next visit.

Postpartum depression checklist

In the past two weeks, how often have you:	A few days	More than half the days	Every day
Felt sad or low?	○	○	○
Felt more tired than usual, or have less energy during the day?	○	○	○
Felt upset or annoyed at little things?	○	○	○
Had trouble thinking, concentrating, or making decisions?	○	○	○
Had no appetite or been eating too much?	○	○	○
Worried that you might hurt yourself or felt like you wanted to die?	○	○	○
Had trouble enjoying things that used to be fun?	○	○	○
Felt like you have no one to talk to?	○	○	○
Felt that you just can't make it through the day?	○	○	○
Felt worthless or hopeless?	○	○	○
Had headaches, backaches, or stomachaches?	○	○	○
Complete the following questions only if you have given birth to a baby in the last 12 months.			
Had problems sleeping when your baby sleeps, or sleeping too much?	○	○	○
Felt numb or disconnected from your baby?	○	○	○
Had scary or negative thoughts about your baby?	○	○	○
Worried that you might hurt your baby?	○	○	○
Felt worried or scared that something bad might happen?	○	○	○
Felt guilty or ashamed about your job as a mom?	○	○	○

APPENDIX B

This is a self-administered questionnaire for patients used to screen for generalized anxiety disorder.

General anxiety disorder seven-item scale

Over the past two weeks, how often have you been bothered by the following problems?	Not at all	Several days	More than half the days	Nearly every day
1. Feeling nervous, anxious, or on edge	0	1	2	3
2. Not being able to stop or control worrying	0	1	2	3
3. Worrying too much about different things	0	1	2	3
4. Having trouble relaxing	0	1	2	3
5. Being so restless that it's hard to sit still	0	1	2	3
6. Becoming easily annoyed or irritable	0	1	2	3
7. Feeling afraid, as if something awful might happen	0	1	2	3
Add the score for each column				
Total score (add your column scores) =				

If you checked off any of the problems, how difficult have these made it for you to do your work, take care of things at home, or get along with other people?

_____ Not difficult at all
_____ Somewhat difficult
_____ Very difficult
_____ Extremely difficult

APPENDIX C: TOP FIVE STRESSORS AND IDEAS FOR TACKLING THEM

List the top five stressors in your life right now. Are those stressors about people, work you have to do, topics you worry about, or a situation that causes emotional reactions? After you've listed the problems, brainstorm ideas for tackling them.

① _____

_____

_____

② _____

_____

_____

③ _____

_____

_____

④ _____

_____

_____

⑤ _____

_____

_____

APPENDIX D: WRITING PROMPTS FOR DISPELLING NEGATIVE THINKING

It is helpful to write out and discharge your ruminations. Get the negative thinking on paper and out of your head. When you're ready, consider the following prompts for promoting a more positive attitude.

What motivates you to keep moving forward?

_____

_____

_____

_____

_____

_____

_____

_____

_____

_____

_____

_____

What makes you happy?

_____

_____

_____

_____

_____

_____

_____

If you could be better at listening to others, how would your life be different?

_____

_____

_____

_____

_____

_____

_____

APPENDIX E: WRITING PROMPTS FOR REFLECTING ON MEANINGFUL MOMENTS

Make a list of the places where you've experienced peace and rejuvenation. Then, you can journey to one enjoyable place in your mind. They'll always be there for you.

Describe your best vacation to a beautiful place or large natural reserve:

_____

_____

_____

Describe your favorite retreat in a garden or park:

_____

_____

_____

List the colors and scents that you like:

_____

_____

_____

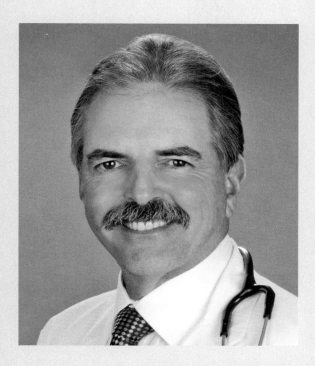

About the Author

Robert S. Rosenberg, D.O., F.C.C.P., is the medical director of the Sleep Disorders Center of Prescott Valley, Arizona, and sleep medicine consultant for Mountain Heart Health Services in Flagstaff, Arizona. Dr. Rosenberg is board-certified in sleep medicine, pulmonary medicine, and internal medicine. He is a contributing sleep expert blogger at EverydayHealth.com, a weekly blogger at Consumer Health Digest, and his advice has appeared in *Women's Health, Prevention, Ladies' Home Journal, Parenting, and O* magazine, among others. Dr. Rosenberg appears on TV, speaks on radio programs, and gives lectures throughout the country on matters concerning sleep medicine.

References

Zhang, Jing, et.al. "Extended Wakefulness: Compromised Metabolics in and Degeneration of Locus Ceruleus Neurons," *The Journal of Neuroscience* 34, no. 12 (2014): 4418–31; doi: 10.1523/JNEUROSCI.5025-12.2014.

Bernal, J. "Night Wakings in Infants during the First 14 Months," *Developmental Medicine & Child Neurology*, no. 15 (1973): 362–72.

Khan, Michal, et al. "Effects of One Night of Induced Night-Wakings versus Sleep Restriction on Sustained Attention and Mood: A Pilot Study," *Sleep Medicine* 15, no. 7 (2014): 825–32. doi:10.1016.

Perelman School of Medicine at the University of Pennsylvania. "Sleeping away infection: Researchers find link between sleep, immune function in fruit flies," Science Daily. www.sciencedaily.com/releases/2014/04/140421211312.htm (accessed June 30, 2015).

Motivala, S. J. et. al. "Inflammatory markers and sleep disturbance in major depression," *Psychosomatic Medicine* 67, (2005): 187-94.

van der Helm, Els, et al. "Sleep Deprivation Impairs the Accurate Recognition of Human Emotions," *Sleep* 33, no. 3 (2010): 335–342.

Patel, Sanjay, et al. "A Prospective Study of Sleep Duration and Pneumonia Risk in Women," *Sleep* 35, no. 1 (2012): 97–101.

Soderquist, F, et al. "Human gastroenteropancreatic expression of melatonin and its receptors MT1 and MT2," *PLoS One* 10, no. 3 (2015): Published online 2015 Mar 30. doi: 10.1371/journal pone.0120195.

Cord, M. J., et al., "Deepening Sleep by Hypnotic Suggestion," *Sleep* 37, no. 6 (2014): 1143–152.

Forster, H.B., et al., "Antispasmodic effects of some medicinal plants," *Planta Medica* 40, (1980): 309–19.

Amsterdam, Jay D. MD. et. al. "A Randomized, Double-Blind, Placebo-Controlled Trial of Oral Matricaria recutita (Chamomile) Extract Therapy for Generalized Anxiety Disorder," *Journal of Clinical Psychopharmacology* 29, no. 4 (2009): 378–82. doi:10.1097/JCP.0b013e3181ac935c.

Elias, N. "Tart Cherry Juice Increases Sleep Time in Older Adults with Insomnia. Experimental Biology," *Journal of Medicinal Food* 13, no. 3 (2010): 579–83. doi:10.1089/jmf.2009.0096.

Kales, A, et al. "Internalization Hypothesis," *Evaluation and Treatment of Insomnia* (1988): 118–22. Accessed January 8, 2015. www.sleep.theclinics.com/article/S1556-407X(07)00047-1/abstract.

Vivek, P., PhD., Roth, T. "Moderators and Mediators of the Relationship between Stress and Insomnia: Stressor Chronicity, Cognitive Intrusion, and Coping," *Sleep* 7, no. 37 (2014): 199–208.

Ong, J. C., et al. "Combining mindfulness meditation with cognitive-behavior therapy for insomnia: A treatment-development study," *Behavioral Therapy* 39, no. 2 (2008): 171–82. doi.10.1016/j.beth.2007.07.002.

Davis, K. "Stress Lies—31 Days of Truth (Day 27)" http://notunredeemed.com/2012/10/27/stress-lies-31-days-of-truth-day-27/#comments. Accessed 1-1-2016.

Arehart-Treichel, J. "Changes in Children's Amygdala Seen after Anxiety Treatment," Anxiety Disorder, Child/Adolescent Psychiatry, *Psychiatric News* 40, no. 9 (2005): 37.

Goldstein, A. N., et al., "Tired and Apprehensive: Anxiety Amplifies the Impact of Sleep Loss on Aversive Brain Anticipation," *Journal of Neuroscience* 33, no. 26 (2013): 10607–615. doi:10.1523/JNEUROSCI.5578-12.2013.

Nader, Karim et al., "Fear memories require protein synthesis in the amygdala for reconsolidation after retrieval," *Nature* 406 (2000): 722–26. doi:10.1038/35021052.

Doyère, V., et.al. "Synapse-specific reconsolidation of distinct fear memories in the lateral amygdala," *Nature Neuroscience* 10, no. 4. (2007): 414–16. doi:10.1038/nn1871.

Krietsch, K. N., et.al. "Sleep complaints predict increases in resting blood pressure following marital separation," *Health Psychology* 33, no. 10 (2014): 1204–13. doi:10.1037/hea0000089. Epub 2014 Jul 14.

Sbarra, David A. et.al. "Marital Dissolution and Blood Pressure Reactivity: Evidence for the Specificity of Emotional Intrusion-Hyperarousal and Task-Rated Emotional Difficulty," *Psychosomatic Medicine* 71, no. 5 (2009): 532–40. doi:10.1097/PSY.0b013e3181a23eee.

Litzelman, Keller A. et al., "Does the perception that stress affects health matter? The association with health and mortality," *Health Psychology* no. 5 (2012): 677–84. doi:10.1037/a0026743. Epub 2011 Dec 26.

Nabi, Hermann., et.al. "Increased risk of coronary heart disease among individuals reporting adverse impact of stress on their health: the Whitehall II prospective cohort study," *European Heart Journal*, no. 34 (2013): 2697–705. doi: 10.1093/eurheartj/eht216.

Morse, D. R., et.al. "Psychosomatically induced death relative to stress, hypnosis, mind control, and voodoo: Review and possible mechanisms," *Stress Medicine*, no. 7 (1991): 213–32.

Poole, Leor J. & Kloner, R. A. "Sudden cardiac death triggered by an earthquake," *New England Journal of Medicine* 334, no. 7 (1996): 413–19.

Gerin, W. et.al., "Sustained blood pressure increase after an acute stressor: The effects of the 11 September 2001 attack on the New York City World Trade Center," *Journal of Hypertension*, no. 23 (2005): 279–84.

Bonanno, G. A. "Loss, trauma, and human resilience: Have we underestimated the human capacity to thrive after extremely aversive events," *American Psychologist*, no. 59 (2004): 20–28.

"Sekiguchi, A, et. al." Resilience after 3/11: structural brain changes 1 year after the Japanese earthquake," *Molecular Psychiatry*, no. 20 (2015): 553–54. doi:10.1038/mp.2014.28; published online April 29, 2014.

Iwadare, Y., et.al. 'Changes in traumatic symptoms and sleep habits among junior high school students after the Great East Japan Earthquake and Tsunami," *Sleep and Biological Rhythms*, no. 12 (2005): 53–61. doi: 10.1111/sbr.12047.

Basta, M., M.D., et.al. "Chronic Insomnia and Stress," *Journal of Clinical Sleep Medicine* 2 no.2 (2007): 279–91.

Marzano, C., et. al. "Quantitative Electroencephalpgram in Insmonia: An New Window on Pathophysiological Mechanisms," *Current Pharmaceutical Designs* 14. no. 14 (2008): 3446–55.

Insomnia Severity Index - My HealtheVet, www.myhealth. va.gov/mhv-portal-web/anonymous.portal?_nfpb=true&_pageLabel=healthyLiving&contentPage=healthy_living/sleep_insomnia_index.htm (accessed June 12, 2015).

Billioti de Gage, Sophie., et al. "Benzodiazepine use and risk of Alzheimer's disease: case-control study," BMJ. 2014; 349 :g5205 BMJ 2014;349:g5205.

Kaestner, Erik J., et.al. "Pharmacologically Increasing Sleep Spindles Enhances Recognition for Negative and High-arousal Memories," *Journal of Cognitive Neuroscience* 25, No. 10 (2013): 1597–1610.

Rodenbeck, A, et. al. "The sleep-improving effects of doxepin are paralleled by a normalized plasma cortisol secretion in primary insomnia. A placebo-controlled, double-blind, randomized, cross-over study followed by an open treatment over 3 weeks," *Psychopharmacology* 170, no. 4 (2003): 423–28.

Wrann, C. D. et al. "Exercise Induces Hippocampal BDNF through a PGC-1/FNDC5 Pathway," *Cell Metabolism* 18, no. 5 (2013): 649–59.

Russo, A.J. "Decreased Zinc and Increased Copper in Individuals with Anxiety," *Nutrition and Metabolic Insights* 4 (2011): 1–5. Accessed January 8, 2015. 10.4137/NMI.S6349.

Southern Methodist University. "Out-of-the-blue panic attacks aren't without warning: Body sends signals for hour before," *ScienceDaily*. www.sciencedaily.com/releases/2011/07/110727122651.htm (accessed June 21, 2015).

Peters, E. M. et., al., "Vitamin C supplementation attenuates the increases in circulating cortisol, adrenaline and anti-inflammatory polypeptides following ultramarathon running," *International Journal of Sports Medicine* 7 (2001): 537–43.

Kiecolt-Glaser, J.K., et. al. "Omega-3 supplementation lowers inflammation and anxiety in medical students: a randomized control trial," *Brain Behavior, and Immunity* 25, no 8. (2011): 1725–34.

Durlach, D., and Bac, P. "Chapter 20: Mechanisms of Action on the Nervous System in Magnesium Deficiency and Dementia," *Mineral and Metal Toxicology*. New York: CRC Press, 1997.

Barbadoro P., et.,al. "Fish oil supplementation reduces cortisol basal levels and perceived stress: a randomized, placebo-controlled trial in abstinent alcoholics." *Molecules Nutrition and Food Research*. 57, no. 6 (2013): 1110–14. doi: 10.1002/mnfr.201200676. Epub 2013 Feb 6.PMID: 23390041.

Trappe, H. J. "Music and health—what kind of music is helpful for whom? What music is not?" *Deutsche Medizinische Wochenschrift* 134, no. 51-52 (2009): 2601–6. doi: 10.1055/s-0029-1243066.

Won, C., and Guilleminault, C. "General Differences in Sleep Disordered Breathing: Implications for Therapy," *Expert Review in Respiratory Medicine* 9, no. 2 (2015): 221–31.

Mavey, P. M., et., al. "Sex Differences in White Matter Alterations Accompanying Obstructive Sleep Apnea, *Sleep* 35, no. 12 (2012): 1603–13.

Rezaeitalab, F., et al. "The Correlation of Anxiety and Depression with Obstructive Sleep Apnea Syndrome," *Journal of Research in Medical Sciences* 19, no. 3 (2014): 205–10. PMID: 24949026.

Tartakovsky, M. (2013) "Depression and Anxiety among College Students," *Psych Central*. Retrieved on June 26, 2015, from http://psychcentral.com/lib/depression-and-anxiety-among-college-students/.

Dark Chocolate Creature | At this stage in my life if it. . . http://darkchocolate-creature.tumblr.com/post/76340682186/at-this-stage-in-my-li (accessed September 06, 2015).

Concha Leo'n-Pizarro, et al. "A randomized trial of the effect of training in relaxation and guided imagery techniques in improving psychological and quality-of-life indices for gynecologic and breast brachytherapy patients, *Psycho-Oncology* 16 (2007): 971–79. doi: 10.1002/pon.1171.

Stahl, James E., Dossett, Michelle L., LaJoie, A. "Relaxation Response and Resiliency Training and its Effect on Healthcare Resource Utilization," *PLoS One*. 2015 October 13, 10.1371.

Hovsepian, Volga, et.al. "A Comparison between Yoga and Aerobic Training Effects on Pulmonary Function Tests and Physical Fitness Parameters," *Pakistan Journal of Medical Sciences* 29, no. 1 (2013): 317–20. http://dx.doi.org/10.12669/pjms.291(Suppl).3524.

P. Chu, R.A., Gotink, G.Y. Yeh, S.J. et. al. "The effectiveness of yoga in modifying risk factors for cardiovascular disease and metabolic syndrome: A systematic review and meta-analysis of randomized controlled trials," *European Journal of Preventive Cardiology* (2014). doi:10.1177/2047487314562741.

Black, David S., et. al. "Yogic meditation reverses NF-κB and IRF-related transcriptome dynamics in leukocytes of family dementia caregivers in a randomized controlled trial." *Psychoneuroendocrinology* 38, no. 3 (2013): 348–55.

Ohio State University. "Yoga can lower fatigue, inflammation in breast cancer survivors," *ScienceDaily*, January 27, 2014. www.sciencedaily.com/releases/2014/01/140127164408.htm.

Richards, Sarah Elizabeth. "4 Science-Backed Ways to Motivate Yourself to Work Out," Huffington Post. www.huffingtonpost.com/2014/09/05/workout-motivation-science_n_5752594.html (accessed July 12, 2015).

Nagendra, Ravindra P., et. al. "Meditation and Its Regulatory Role on Sleep," *Frontiers in Neurology* 3 (2012): 54. doi:10.3389/fneur.2012.00054. Web. 2 July 2015.

Wallace, R. K., "Physiological effects of transcendental meditation." *Revista Brasileira de Medicina*. Med. 8, (1970): 397–401.

Sulekha, S., et. al., "Evaluation of sleep architecture in practitioners of Sudarshan Kriya yoga and Vipassana meditation," *Sleep and Biological Rhythms* 4, no. 3 (2006): 207–14. dio:10.1111/j.1479-8425.2006.00233.x.

Nagendra, Ravindra P. et. al., "Practitioners of Vipassana meditation exhibit enhanced slow wave sleep and REM sleep states across different age groups." *Sleep and Biological Rhythms* 8, no. 1 (2010): 34–41. doi: 10.1111/j.1479-8425.2009.00416.x.

Infante, J. R., et. al., "Catecholamine levels in practitioners of the transcendental meditation technique," *Physiology and Behavior* 72 (2001): 141–6.

Bratman, Gregory R., et.al "The Benefits of Nature Experience: improved affect and cognition," *Landscape and Urban Planning* 138, (2015) 41–50.

Marselle, Melissa R., Ph.D., M.Sc., et.al. "Examining group walks in nature and multiple aspects of well-being: A large scale study," *Ecopsychology* 6, no. 3 (2014): 134–47. doi: 10.1089/eco.2014.0027.

Rizic, A. et al., "Regular Dog-walking Improves Physical Capacity in Elderly Patients after Myocardial Infarction," *Collegium Antropolgicum* 25, no. 2 (2011): 73–5.

"A Modern Use for an Ancient Skill," Cancer-MN Health Center: Article: http://MotherNature.com. Accessed July 26, 2015. www.mothernature.com/archive.

Pennebaker, James W., et.al. "Disclosure of Traumas and Immune Function: Health Implications for Psychotherapy," *Journal of Consulting and Clinical Psychology* 56, no. 2 (1998): 239–45. Accessed August 3, 2015. doi:10.1037/0022-006x.56.2.239.

Index